Gastroenterology

Editor

TRACEY K. RITZMAN

VETERINARY CLINICS OF NORTH AMERICA: EXOTIC ANIMAL PRACTICE

www.vetexotic.theclinics.com

Consulting Editor
AGNES E. RUPLEY

May 2014 • Volume 17 • Number 2

ELSEVIER

1600 John F. Kennedy Boulevard ● Suite 1800 ● Philadelphia, Pennsylvania, 19103-2899
http://www.vetexotic.theclinics.com

VETERINARY CLINICS OF NORTH AMERICA: EXOTIC ANIMAL PRACTICE Volume 17, Number 2
May 2014 ISSN 1094-9194, ISBN-13: 978-0-323-29727-1

Editor: Patrick Manley
Developmental Editor: Casey Jackson

Veterinary Clinics of North America: Exotic Animal Practice (ISSN 1094-9194) is published in January, May, and September by Elsevier, Inc., 360 Park Avenue South, New York, NY 10010-1710. Subscription prices are $255.00 per year for US individuals, $399.00 per year for US institutions, $130.00 per year for US students and residents, $305.00 per year for Canadian individuals, $482.00 per year for Canadian institutions, $340.00 per year for international individuals, $482.00 per year for international institutions and $165.00 per year for Canadian and foreign students/residents. To receive student/resident rate, orders must be accompanied by name of affiliated institution, date of term, and the *signature* of program/residency coordinator on institution letterhead. Orders will be billed at individual rate until proof of status is received. Foreign air speed delivery is included in all *Clinics* subscription prices. All prices are subject to change without notice. **POSTMASTER:** Send address changes to *Veterinary Clinics of North America: Exotic Animal Practice*, Elsevier Health Sciences Division, Subscription Customer Service, 3251 Riverport Lane, Maryland Heights, MO 63043. **Customer Service: Telephone: 1-800-654-2452** (U.S. and Canada); **1-314-447-8871** (outside U.S. and Canada). **Fax: 1-314-447-8029. E-mail: journalscustomerservice-usa@elsevier.com** (for print support); **journalsonlinesupport-usa@elsevier.com** (for online support).

Reprints. For copies of 100 or more of articles in this publication, please contact the Commercial Reprints Department, Elsevier Inc., 360 Park Avenue South, New York, New York 10010-1710. Tel.: 212-633-3874; Fax: 212-633-3820; E-mail: reprints@elsevier.com.

Veterinary Clinics of North America: Exotic Animal Practice is covered in *MEDLINE/PubMed (Index Medicus)*.

Contributors

CONSULTING EDITOR

AGNES E. RUPLEY, DVM
Diplomate, American Board of Veterinary Practitioners–Avian Practice; Director and Chief Veterinarian, All Pets Medical & Laser Surgical Center, College Station, Texas

EDITOR

TRACEY K. RITZMAN, DVM
Diplomate, American Board of Veterinary Practitioners-Avian and Exotic Companion Mammal; Cascade Hospital for Animals, Grand Rapids, Michigan

AUTHORS

JESSICA BASSECHES, DVM
Diplomate of the American College of Veterinary Radiologists; Center for Animal Referral and Emergency Services, Langhorne, Pennsylvania

RYAN S. DE VOE, DVM, MSpVM
Diplomate of the American College of Zoological Medicine; Diplomate of the American Board of Veterinary Practitioners (Avian); Diplomate of the American Board of Veterinary Practitioners (Reptile and Amphibian); Senior Veterinarian, North Carolina Zoological Park, Asheboro, North Carolina

JENNIFER GRAHAM, DVM
Diplomate of the American Board of Veterinary Practitioners (Avian/Exotic Companion Mammal); Diplomate of the American College of Zoological Medicine; Assistant Professor, Department of Zoological Companion Animal Medicine, Cummings School of Veterinary Medicine, Tufts University, North Grafton, Massachusetts; Affiliate Assistant Professor, Department of Comparative Medicine, University of Washington School of Medicine, Seattle, Washington

BARBARA HEIDENREICH, BS Zoology
Good Bird Inc, Austin, Texas

MICAH KOHLES, DVM, MPA
Oxbow Animal Health; School of Veterinary Medicine and Biomedical Sciences, University of Nebraska-Lincoln, Nebraska, Nebraska

ADOLF K. MAAS III, DVM
Diplomate of the American Board of Veterinary Practitioners (Reptile and Amphibian Practice); ZooVet Consulting, PLLC, Bothell, Washington

MAUREEN MURRAY, DVM
Diplomate, American Board of Veterinary Practitioners-Avian Practice; Clinical Assistant Professor, Wildlife Clinic, Tufts Cummings School of Veterinary Medicine, North Grafton, Massachusetts

DAVID N. PHALEN, DVM, PhD
Diplomate of the American Board of Veterinary Practitioners (Avian); Associate Professor, Faculty of Veterinary Science, University of Sydney, Camden, New South Wales, Australia

DRURY REAVILL, DVM
Diplomate American Board of Veterinary Practitioners (Avian and Reptile & Amphibian Practice); Diplomate American College of Veterinary Pathologists; Zoo/Exotic Pathology Service, West Sacramento, California

TRACEY K. RITZMAN, DVM
Diplomate, American Board of Veterinary Practitioners-Avian and Exotic Companion Mammal; Cascade Hospital for Animals, Grand Rapids, Michigan

E. SCOTT WEBER III, VMD, MSc
Science and Technology Policy Fellow, American Association for the Advancement of Science, Washington, DC; Adjunct Clinical Professor, Veterinary Medicine and Epidemiology, UC Davis School of Veterinary Medicine, Davis, California

Contents

for ileus include fluid therapy, pain relief, nutritional support, and prokinetic therapy. The prognosis of the exotic mammal patient with gastrointestinal disease depends on the timing of the diagnosis and initiation of treatment. Surgical conditions such as gastrointestinal obstruction can have a good outcome if diagnosed early.

This article reviews diagnosis and management of liver lobe torsion in rabbits. Practitioners should recommend initial diagnostics including radiographs and blood work on rabbits presenting with nonspecific signs of gastrointestinal (GI) stasis to better determine possible etiology and make the best treatment recommendations. If hepatic enzyme elevation is found in a rabbit with GI stasis, abdominal ultrasound is recommended to rule out liver lobe torsion. Prompt diagnosis and liver lobectomy are recommended for best outcome in rabbits with liver lobe torsion.

Macrorhabdus ornithogaster, a yeast found only at the junction between the ventriculus and proventriculus, can infect a wide range of birds. Infection is often subclinical but can also result in gastrointestinal signs. Direct observation of the organism in the feces is a specific but somewhat insensitive means of diagnosis. At least three antifungal drugs are reported to be effective for treatment but resistance to one or more of these drugs may occur.

Free-living raptors are frequently presented to wildlife rehabilitation centers. Conditions affecting the gastrointestinal tract can be the primary reason for presentation. The gastrointestinal tract can also be affected secondary to debilitation from other injuries or from the stress of the rehabilitation process. A thorough understanding of the anatomy, physiology, and natural history of these species is crucial to successful treatment and rehabilitation. This article addresses raptor gastroenterology with an emphasis on conditions affecting free-living birds.

 Video of guinea pig motivated to climb onto a scale; aviary birds motivated for training; managed delivery of a skunk's regular diet; Macaw with free access to pelleted food; and a rabbit calm and relaxed for nail trimming accompany this article

Food plays an important part in companion animal health, and also plays a significant role in influencing animal behavior. Avian and small mammal species show general trends in food preferences that can be used to reinforce desired behaviors. Motivation for food can be increased by various strategies. Nonfood reinforcers also offer additional options for reinforcing behaviors when food is of little value to an animal. Transitioning to less rich, healthier diets can help prevent reproductive hormone amplification. This article explores how delivering food is an opportunity to influence behavior in addition to providing nourishment.

Providing nutritional support to reptile patients is a challenging and often misunderstood task. Ill reptiles are frequently anorexic and can benefit greatly from appropriate nutrition delivered via a variety of assist-feeding techniques. Neonatal reptiles can also be very challenging patients because many fail to thrive without significant efforts to establish normal feeding behaviors. This article presents ideas supporting the benefit of timely nutritional support as well as specific recommendations for implementation of assist feeding. Also discussed are a few nutritional issues that affect captive reptile species.

In mammals, gastrointestinal protozoal organism inhabitation has been well-studied, with hundreds of species defined as parasites. While the mammalian protozoal relationships have been identified and categorized by anatomy, tropism, pathogenicity, and life cycles, relatively few species of protozoal organism relationships have been categorized in reptiles. Species of parasites are still being segregated from each other, and conflicting information needs to be clarified to completely understand the data already available. This article presents the information available to help reptile practitioners make evidence-based decisions regarding both the determination of a pathologic parasitic condition and direct appropriate treatment of patients.

VETERINARY CLINICS OF NORTH AMERICA: EXOTIC ANIMAL PRACTICE

RELATED INTEREST

Veterinary Clinics of North America: Small Animal Practice,
March 2011 (Vol. 41, No. 6)
Chronic Intestinal Diseases of Dogs and Cats
Frédéric P. Gaschen, Dr med vet, Dr habil, *Editor*

THE CLINICS ARE NOW AVAILABLE ONLINE!
Access your subscription at:
www.theclinics.com

Preface

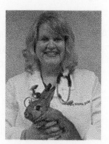

Tracey K. Ritzman, DVM, Diplomate ABVP-Avian & Exotic
Companion Mammal
Editor

The common saying "time flies" certainly applies to the time between when the first issue of *Veterinary Clinics of North America: Exotic Animal Practice*, focused on gastroenterology for exotic pets, was published in May of 2005 and this edition for 2014. Over those nine years a great deal has been learned and accomplished in the field of veterinary medicine for exotic animal patients. During this timeframe, our profession has seen several new species-specific specialties come to fruition through the American Board of Veterinary Practitioners in both Reptile and Amphibian and Exotic Companion Mammal practice categories. I expect those of you reading this message can quickly think about this timeframe and recall certain events in your lives, both personal and professional, of importance during those years! Gastroenterology continues to be a prominent topic for veterinary clinicians today.

The purpose of this issue is to provide an update to the veterinary clinician and animal care professionals on current topics in gastroenterology of avian, reptilian, amphibian, piscine, and exotic companion mammal patients. Just as in the human medical field, gastroenterology remains a dynamic, prominent, and continuously evolving area of medicine and surgery. This publication provides an interesting combination of anatomy, physiology, medicine, and surgery articles pertaining to gastroenterology.

I am very fortunate to have a great group of authors from geographical areas throughout the United States as well as from other countries contributing to this issue. The authors are all very dedicated to the veterinary profession and the care and wellness of the animals in their lives. I am honored to be a guest editor for this topic for a second time. I extend my sincere gratitude for the time, efforts, and sacrifices the authors have made in contributing to this publication.

Vet Clin Exot Anim 17 (2014) ix–x
http://dx.doi.org/10.1016/j.cvex.2014.02.001
1094-9194/14/$ – see front matter © 2014 Elsevier Inc. All rights reserved.

vetexotic.theclinics.com

A thank you also, to the Elsevier staff, including Casey Jackson, Patrick Manley, and John Vassallo, who provided their support, knowledge, and skills to bring this publication to print.

Tracey K. Ritzman, DVM, Diplomate ABVP-Avian & Exotic Companion Mammal
Cascade Hospital for Animals
6730 Cascade Road, S.E.
Grand Rapids, MI 49546, USA
http://chfa.net

E-mail address:
tritzman@chfa.net

A Veterinary Guide to the Fish Gastrointestinal Tract

E. Scott Weber III, VMD, MSc[a,b,*]

KEYWORDS

- Gastrointestinal tract • Gastroscopy • Buoyancy disorder • Taurine deficiency
- Prebiotics • Probiotics • Thiaminase

KEY POINTS

- Advanced diagnostic techniques can be practically modified and directly applied to fish patients for identifying gastrointestinal ailments.
- Prebiotics and probiotics may treat and prevent infectious diseases, enhance oral medication and vaccine uptake, and can better maintain healthy and normal gastrointestinal flora in fish.
- More research investigating the normal intestinal flora of fish, oral pharmacokinetics for both drugs and vaccines, optimal nutritional requirements for various species, and the role of mucosal immunity on protection against common fish pathogens serves to improve the veterinary approach for a broader and more comprehensive understanding of fish gastroenterology.

Key objectives

- Expand on veterinary comparative anatomic knowledge of the fish gastrointestinal tract
- Show through case management the use of modern diagnostic tools for identifying gastrointestinal problems in fish patients such as dysphagia and buoyancy disorder
- Introduce additional concepts of veterinary gastroenterology concerns regarding the piscine patient regarding toxins, nutritional deficiencies, prebiotics and probiotics, and zoonotic agents
- Update differential chart with specific infectious disease examples

---

INTRODUCTION

Gastroenterology in osteichthyes (bony fishes), which comprise most species of veterinary concern, such as salmon, koi, and catfish, and in chondrichthyes

---

[a] AAAS, 1200 New York Avenue Northwest, Washington, DC 20005, USA; [b] Veterinary Medicine and Epidemiology, 2108 Tupper Hall, UC Davis School of Veterinary Medicine, Davis, CA 95616, USA
* 162 Greenfields Lane, White Post, VA 22663.
E-mail address: Sharkdoc01@gmail.com

Vet Clin Exot Anim 17 (2014) 123–143
http://dx.doi.org/10.1016/j.cvex.2014.01.001
1094-9194/14/$ – see front matter © 2014 Elsevier Inc. All rights reserved.

(cartilaginous fishes), which include sharks, rays, and skates, continues to be a growing area for research and new clinical treatments.[1] Advanced diagnostic techniques can be practically modified and directly applied to fish patients for identifying gastrointestinal ailments. Prebiotics and probiotics may treat and prevent infectious diseases, could enhance oral medication and vaccine uptake, and can better maintain healthy and normal gastrointestinal flora in fish. More research investigating the normal intestinal flora of fish, oral pharmacokinetics for both drugs and vaccines, optimal nutritional requirements for various species, and the role of mucosal immunity on protection against common fish pathogens serves to improve the veterinary approach for a broader and more comprehensive understanding of fish gastroenterology.

Although no unique veterinary specialty is recognized for fish medicine or aquatic animal health in the United States, veterinarians have been expanding their experience, increasing their knowledge, and contributing to the veterinary literature for the last several decades to advance medicine and surgery for aquatic vertebrates and invertebrates. Several professional organizations have been created to support aquatic veterinarians, including the American Association of Fish Veterinarians, the World Aquatic Veterinary Medical Association, and the International Association of Aquatic Animal Medicine.

There are 3 extant classes of fish, which include agnatha (jawless fishes), chondrichthyes, and osteichthyes, with 60,229 described species and subspecies, and 32,590 species scientifically validated.[2–4] Clinically, veterinarians may serve or consult with a wide variety of clients, including hobbyists or pet owners, laboratory researchers, pet and pharmaceutical industries, fisheries managers, public aquaria and zoologic gardens, public health, ornamental aquaria aquaculture, mariculture, and food production aquaculture. When presented with morbidity or mortality of an individual animal or population, often, a thorough medical history can provide invaluable information for making an expedient diagnosis; for population health, a quick diagnosis is critical for managing disease outbreaks, which can cause catastrophically high morbidity/mortality.

THE PISCINE GASTROINTESTINAL TRACT

Fish comprise the 3 largest extant classes of vertebrates, and, given the great diversity across these classes, comparative similarities and differences in the piscine gastrointestinal tract are highlighted. For veterinarians to better understand aquatic animal health, the most basic veterinary foundation begins with understanding fish anatomy and physiology.

The piscine gastrointestinal tract begins with apprehension of food through the teeth, mouth, and pharynx, and then progresses down the esophagus, stomach, intestines, and pyloric ceca, with waste elimination out the cloacae, vent, or anus. The liver, pancreas, and gallbladder are vital to digestion, as in other vertebrates. Although the swim bladder has a role in buoyancy control for many teleost species, embryologically, it is derived from the esophagus.[1]

OVERVIEW OF ANATOMY

Some of the earliest comprehensive works on understanding the gross anatomic and histologic differences of the gastrointestinal tract in fish were published in the 1930s. This series of research compared the gastrointestinal tracts of bottom-dwelling, predaceous, and planktivorous fishes. The following sections highlight anatomic differences among these groups.

GENERAL ANATOMIC DIFFERENCES OF BOTTOM-FEEDER SEA ROBIN (*PRIONOTUS CAROLINUS*)

Sea robins opportunistically ingest whole prey items that drift past them on the bottom of the ocean, bay, or estuary.[5] Because of this feeding strategy, this species has a wide mouth, leading to a short esophagus, consisting of a muscular layer, connective tissue layer, and mucosal layers, analogous to other fish and vertebrates.[5] The stomach of *Prionotus carolinus* is tubular and has a pyloric cecal arrangement, conserved in other gurnard fish from this group.[6] Grossly, the pyloric verses cardiac areas of the stomach are indistinguishable, but on histopathology, the large cardiac region consists of secreting gastric or peptic cells.[5] Similar species in this grouping such as the monkfish (*Lophius americanus*), can ingest greater than 50% of their body weight at a single feeding, whereas other nonrelated fishes, like tetras, Characidae, have smaller stomach capacities, which hold roughly 10% of body weight. In a previous Veterinary Clinics issue, a radiograph of a sea raven (*Hemitripterus americanus*), after ingesting a lead weight shows the indiscriminate feeding behavior of this group.[1] The intestine of these animals is roughly 3 to 5 times body length, with 3 distinct areas, the foremost being pyloric cecae.[5] These fish have a delineated liver, pancreas, and gallbladder.

The liver in most fish is found in the anterior abdomen and can be a large discrete organ or can appear more disseminated, intimately associated in adipose tissue along loops of intestine or pyloric ceca. The pancreas grossly may appear as a discrete organ, or be diffusely found in the liver, only evident as discrete pancreatic tissue histologically. Although sometimes referred to by the misnomer hepatopancreas, this organ is not the same hepatopancreas as invertebrates, because in fish there is a true differentiation of pancreatic versus hepatic tissue when viewed microscopically. Unlike other vertebrates, histologic sectioning of the liver in fish does not show distinct chords and lobes, but rather consists of sinusoids that are distinguished by a separation of blood and bile on opposite sides. Lipid accumulation, especially for captive reared fish from a variety of sources, can abundantly occur in the hepatocytes; this hepatic lipidosis may or may not be a pathologic finding, depending on the nutrition, husbandry, species, and medical history for these animals. As a histologic example, shark hepatocytes normally have tremendous lipid accumulation caused by the production of squalene for buoyancy control, whereas this same appearance for a *Prionotus carolinus*, sea bass (*Centropristes striatus*), or minnow (*Campostoma anomalum*) liver most likely would indicate some underlying disease. Fish can survive extensive liver necrosis compared with mammals, birds, and reptiles, because of hepatic regeneration, and hepatic toxicity in fish lacks the presence of zonal cell death or necrosis patterns observed in other vertebrates.[7]

GENERAL ANATOMIC DIFFERENCES OF PREDACEOUS SEA BASS (*CENTROPRISTES STRIATUS*)

The pharynx is not well differentiated in these animals, and this piscivorous species has a muscular short esophagus, leading to a J-shaped stomach, which is highly distensible.[8] Comparatively, stomach anatomy in fish can range from the presence of an intestinal bulb to a thick-walled gizzardlike organ found in certain surgeon fishes, Acanthuridae. The stomach in many predatory or piscivorous fish species is sigmoidal or J-shaped, highly distensible, and possesses significant folds, which form multiple rugae. In several species of fish, blind-ended pouches or diverticula numbering from 2 to more than a thousand called pyloric ceca are located at the pyloric valve near the duodenum. The gastric portion of the stomach is marked by an increase in numerous glands at the base of the folds, resembling chief cells in other vertebrates, and some gastric glands also contain tubules, which contain zymogen-like secretory granules, which are released by exocytosis, similar to oxyntic cells found in higher vertebrates.[8] Chemical digestion occurs in the stomach in many fish. Some animals depend on acid production to create a low pH environment, similar to other vertebrates, to activate enzymatic cascades for food breakdown. Gastric glands in the stomach produce pepsin, but other enzymes produced in the stomach have also been described. Pepsin and low pH are primarily responsible for the chemical digestion of food, especially in highly predatory species of fish. Digestion and absorption of nutrients sequentially continues in the pyloric ceca, which have mucoid columnar epithelial cells devoid of villi. The intestine in these piscivorous or carnivorous animals is short, leading from pyloric cecae to anus, compared with the sea robin and minnow.

GENERAL ANATOMIC AND HISTOLOGIC DIFFERENCES OF PLANKTONIC MINNOW (*CAMPOSTOMA ANOMALUM*)

The pharynx of this species is divided into anterior and posterior, with callous raised pads referred to as pharyngeal teeth located in the posterior pharynx, a unique anatomic feature when compared with the bottom-feeding sea robin and predaceous sea bass.[9] The anterior pharynx is the only location of a true stratum compactum in the gastrointestinal tract of the minnow, whereas in predatory fish, such as salmon, the stratum compactum is found throughout the gastrointestinal tract.[10] Paired flask-shaped taste buds are found in submucosal papilla from the pharynx down to the esophagus of *Campostoma anomalum*.[9] Unlike in the sea robin and bass, the minnow lacks a true stomach and has an intestinal bulb lacking any of the peptic or gastric glands described in the stomachs of other fishes. The length of the intestine varies in fish, similar to higher vertebrates, with carnivorous animals having short tracts and herbivorous fishes having long coiled intestinal tracts. Herbivorous fish often have intestines up to 20 times the length of the animal's body. Carnivorous fish, such as the sea bass, often have a very short digestive tract (one-fifth of body length), often only as long as the distance between the mouth and anus, as seen in trout, Salmonidae. The intestines terminate near the ventrocaudal area of the fish through the anus, or empty into a cloaca, which serves as a small vestibule for excretion of the digestive waste, urinary waste, and reproductive products through the vent. Gastrointestinal motility is supported by smooth muscle contraction of the intestinal walls, with dietary and environmental factors (water, temperature, season) dictating gastrointestinal transit time for a specific species.[9] An interesting clinical finding found in several species of fish including predatory and plankitorous animals (8 cases) has been the strangulation of intestines and disruption of buoyancy control caused by intracoelomic lipomas. These lipomas often cannot be surgically removed and intimately surround the posterior gastrointestinal tract (**Fig. 1**).

GENERAL ONTOGENY
Digestion and Absorption

Many of the digestive enzymes occurring in other vertebrates are also present in fish. Some enzymes characterized from fish have both proteolytic and amylase activities, including amylase, cellulase, invertase, esterase, and acid and alkaline proteases, with production taking place in the esophagus, stomach, intestines, or liver.[11]

In other vertebrates, these proteolytic and amylase enzymes have activity and production that are often limited to specific anatomic locations in the gastrointestinal tract, and enzyme abundance and activity is specifically related to dietary habits

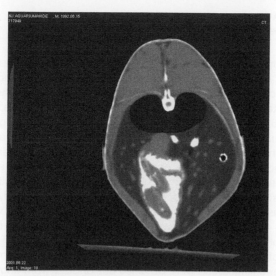

Fig. 1. A transverse computer-assisted tomography scan section through the anterior coelom of a largemouth bass (*Micropterus salmoides*) showing a lipomatous mass (*contrast*) strangulating the intestines. This mass was inoperable and the animal had to be euthanized because it could no longer maintain proper orientation in the water column.

and food preference. Chakrabarti and colleagues[11] investigated different enzyme production in 11 different species of freshwater fish to identify effects of these enzymes based on species food preferences and food niche segregation.[11] The findings suggested that enzyme production for both amylase and protease activity is maintained throughout the gastrointestinal tract and does not seem restricted based on segregation of food niche, preference, or habit. Developmental research in marine larval fish found that diet composition can enhance, stop, or delay functional development of specific digestive enzymes.[12]

Immunology

Several fish species such as tuna or thunnis (Scombridae) have an abundant amount of gastrointestinal-associated lymphoid tissue, which can be confused histologically with disease processes when reviewing fish histopathology slides for the first time.

Some of the research specific for fish gut-associated lymphoid tissue has included understanding the basic cell identity, cell population, and structure of these lymphoid aggregates; investigating how these cell populations are involved with absorption of various macromolecules from the intestinal lumen; and identifying the production and composition of specific mucosal antibodies in relation to antigen uptake.[13] The fish gastrointestinal role in immunology relies greatly on the innate immune system and there is a general lack of leukocyte-rich Peyer patches such as in mammals. In most fish, populations of leukocytes are found in the lamina propria of the intestinal rugae, and smaller populations are intraepithelial; the degree, extent, and amount of these leukocyte populations vary with species.[14] From the perspective of aquatic animal health, the ability of fish to absorb bioactive proteins and macromolecules through their gastrointestinal tract provides impetus for development and research into orally administered fish pharmaceuticals and vaccines to help prevent and control outbreaks of infectious disease.[15]

DIFFERENTIAL DIAGNOSIS
Noninfectious: Dietary Indiscretion Case

Medical history

A client-owned adult wolf fish (*Hoplias aimara*), wild captured from the tributaries of the middle and lower Amazon basin, was presented with a history of anorexia, vomiting, and listing from side to side. Although this animal had been in captivity for 2 to 3 years, the fish was maintained in its present conditions for the last 6 months. The animal was housed in a 1818-L (400-gallon) freshwater aquarium with a pea gravel substrate. Water quality results indicated increased ammonia (0.05–0.30 ppm) and nitrate levels (15–20 ppm); both can lead to anorexia, acute and chronic gill disease, nonspecific chronic associated health problems, or death. Nutritional husbandry exclusively relied on feeding pieces of frozen river smelt (*Thaleichthys pacificus*), with an infrequent addition of live oscars (*Astronotus ocellatus*). *Hoplias aimara* is rarely held by private hobbyists, because it is a large nocturnal carnivore; the heaviest weight recorded for this species is 40 kg, and it has several rows of razor-sharp teeth for prey capture. The medical history of this animal included the per os administration of pieces of fish injected with enrofloxacin calculated using an anecdotal dosage without dosed using the animal's weight. Antibiotics were obtained out-of-state from another veterinarian via phone consultation only.

Physical examination

On presentation, the fish was bright, alert, and responsive, with a body length of 78.7 cm (31 in) and mass of 7.7 kg. The animal was left laterally recumbent and unable to maintain an upright normal posture in the water column, despite attempting to right itself periodically. Based on the physical examination findings, further diagnostics were recommended, which included a general physical examination, radiography, ultrasonography, parasitology, and hematology.

MEDICAL/SURGICAL PROCEDURES
Anesthesia

Anesthesia was maintained using a bath of MS-222 (Finquel Argent Laboratories) at 75 ppm buffered with 35 ppm of sodium bicarbonate; chemicals were added directly into 75 L of water containing the fish, and because this animal was from a region with acidic water quality conditions, only half the amount of sodium bicarbonate (Arm & Hammer) normally used was added as a buffer to reduce the acidity of the MS-222. Confining this large freshwater animal to 75 L may also have an unintended consequence of ammonia accumulation during the procedure because of gill respiration, so maintaining a lower pH can also serve to shift ammonia to a chemically favorable nontoxic ammonium state in water. Air was supplied to the water with an air stone attached to a standard aquarium air pump.

Radiography and Ultrasonography

An ultrasound scan was performed on the coelom to look for potential gastrointestinal or gonadal masses. The animal had digital radiography, followed by a contrast study using iodinated contrast. Dorsoventral and horizontal beam lateral radiographs were performed, showing an unidentified foreign body using a kVp = 70, mA = 400, and mAs = 5 technique optimized for survey and contrast radiography. A horizontal beam lateral radiograph is commonly used in fish and allows for the coelomic organs to remain in normal anatomic position; this technique provides better soft tissue contrast in the coelomic cavity, especially when the coelom is distended from ascites. A gastrointestinal contrast study was performed using 60 mL of iodinated contrast agent by mouth via an 18-gauge French rubber catheter inserted into the mouth and advanced to the level of the stomach, as estimated based on the survey films, and then contrast (15–20 mL) was given retrograde by advancing an 18-gauge French rubber catheter through the vent and into the intestines.

Diagnosis

On the survey radiographs, there was a radiopacity similar to mineral density within the ventral coelomic cavity shaped like a half sphere (**Fig. 2**). On contrast radiography, the gastrogram showed the foreign body within the stomach, although no evidence of a blockage in the intestinal tract was observed from the retrograde administration of contrast given via enema. From observations on the contrast radiographs, important anatomically information was obtained for this species regarding the presence of a large pouchlike stomach, similar to other predatory fish species, which empties cranially and dorsally into a very narrow intestine, which is about one-fifth the body length of this animal. This gastrointestinal anatomy created a situation for a foreign body to act as a ball valve between the stomach and the duodenum, allowing food to enter the stomach but then preventing food from moving into the intestines via peristalsis, resulting in the observed clinical signs. Based on these findings, the client was advised that this animal would require endoscopy or surgery to remove the ingested foreign body.

Endoscopy

Endoscopy is a valuable diagnostic tool for fish patients, similar to mammals, birds, reptiles, and amphibians. Endoscopes can be used in fish patients to perform oral and opercular examinations, gastroscopy, colonoscopy, and celioscopy. In some cases, when fish are poor candidates for longer coelomic surgery, endoscopy may offer an option for obtaining biopsies and gathering vital diagnostic information.[16]

To maintain anesthesia, the fish was placed in ventral recumbency contained in a large plastic trough on a surgical table, and fenestrated sylastic tubing was placed into the right and left gills of the fish through the mouth and held in place using a 20-mL syringe inserted into the end of tubing protruding from each gill operculum (**Fig. 3**). Water containing the anesthetic was then pumped through the tubes using a submersible power head pump to provide anesthesia and assist the fish with respiration. The heart rate of the fish was monitored using a Doppler during the procedure.

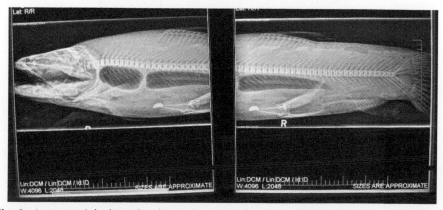

Fig. 2. A survey right lateral radiograph using a horizontal beam showing a radiopaque semicircular crescent-shaped foreign body in the stomach of a *Hoplias aimara*.

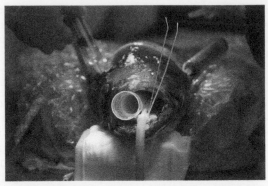

Fig. 3. *Hoplias aimara* under general anesthesia being prepared for gastric endoscopy. Note the gills are being constantly bathed with an anesthetic bath via a continuous pump and supported using syringes. The 60-mL syringe case placed in the oral cavity was used to protect the endoscope from extensive dentition.

A 60-mL syringe case with its closed end cut off was secured in the mouth of the fish to protect the endoscope. A flexible 5.0-mm endoscope with 2.9-mm channel and video camera was used for this procedure (Karl Storz Endoscopy, Goleta, CA). Once the endoscope was placed down the esophagus and into the stomach, the foreign body was quickly found and identified as a stone (**Fig. 4**). A 2.5-FR 120-cm stone wire basket tool was placed through the port and the stone was easily captured and removed (Karl Storz). The stone was a piece of the pea gravel substrate that measured 3.1 cm long × 1.2 cm wide × 0.6 cm deep (**Fig. 5**). After the procedure, on recovery from anesthesia, the animal regained normal body posture and no longer was left laterally recumbent or struggling to right itself.

Endoscopy and celioscopy in poikilotherms is becoming a more common practice for both diagnostic and treatment applications. In fish, celioscopy has been used in

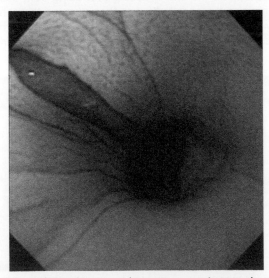

Fig. 4. A still image from the endoscopy video capture equipment showing a stone in the stomach of a *Hoplias aimara*.

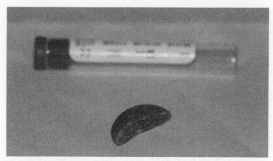

Fig. 5. A piece of pea gravel aquarium substrate removed from the stomach of a *Hoplias aimara* using gastroscopy.

field research to successfully sex both male and female gulf sturgeon and rainbow trout.[17,18] Celioscopy is also being used to obtain diagnostic tissue biopsies from gonads, liver, and spleen in brook trout for histopathology (Charles Innis, personal communication, 2007). Endoscopy has several other applications in fish medicine and as shown provides less invasive treatment modalities for common problems that can occur in fish patients.[16]

SUMMARY

The medical history for this animal raised several veterinary questions and ethical dilemmas specific for this patient pertaining to adequately sized habitat, properly decorated habitat, natural history of species, ideal diet for genus, possible dietary deficiencies, optimal husbandry required, acceptable water and environmental quality, animal welfare concerns, and appropriate and legal treatment using antibiotics. These questions pose additional challenges for incorporating aquatic animals into a small animal practice, and during an on-site visit to monitor recovery of this animal, these questions were addressed over several months through frank client/veterinary discussions. This case also shows how advanced diagnostic techniques and equipment for digital radiography, ultrasonography, and endoscopy can be easily applied for use in fish patients.

BUOYANCY DISORDERS

The most common clinical presentation of fancy goldfish (*Carassius auratus auratus*) brought into the veterinary hospital is buoyancy disorders. These disorders have a wide range of clinical presentations of animals being negatively or positively buoyant, listing from side to side, lacking a righting reflex, or appearing with the craniad or caudad oriented head downward or tail dragging. The cause of buoyancy disorders in goldfish can populate a differential list, with the most common being infectious disease of the swim bladder, gastrointestinal, renal, or reproductive tract caused by primary or secondary bacterial, fungal, viral, or myxozoan infections, tumors, trauma, toxins, or idiopathic.[19] Advanced diagnostic imaging can assist in isolating the appropriate organ system affected.[20,21] Polycystic kidney disease and coelomic tumors are easily distinguished using ultrasonography, digital radiography, and computed tomography (computer-assisted tomography scan) (**Fig. 6**).[22–25] Two common clinical presentations radiographically can show primary swim bladder involvement, either hyperinflated or hypoinflated, or it may appear as a gas-distended intestine, similar

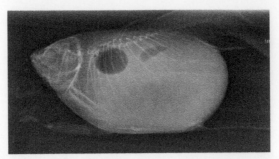

Fig. 6. Right lateral radiograph of a goldfish diagnosed with polycystic kidney disease. Note that the caudal swim bladder chamber is reduced in size and displaced ventrally away from the spinal column. (*Courtesy of* Dr Lori Campbell, University of California at Davis Veterinary Teaching Hospital, Davis, CA.)

to presentation in other animals as an intestinal obstruction (**Figs. 7** and **8**). Many cases with primary swim bladder involvement prove to be idiopathic, and several cases marked by a dilated gastrointestinal tract are an intestinal pseudo-obstruction, rather than true gastrointestinal obstructions. The causes of these 2 latter presentations of idiopathic buoyancy disorder caused by a malfunctioning swim bladder or intestinal pseudo-obstruction need further investigation. The causes of intestinal pseudo-obstruction in other animals, including humans, are genetic defects, smooth muscle myopathy, neurologic disorders, associated secondarily with other degenerative diseases, trauma, renal insufficiency, hypothyroidism, severe constipation, several cancers, and iatrogenically, with several types of medications.[26–28] This syndrome has also been reported in fish.[29] Because breeding for these goldfish varieties is based solely on color and unusual body conformation, a prevailing theory that could explain both these syndromes based on genetic disposition and conformation is a secondary neuropathy related to spinal cord trauma. The swim bladder evaginates from the intestines, and in this species, forms a pneumoduct connecting the swim bladder to the esophagus.[30] A neuropathy may develop affecting either the swim

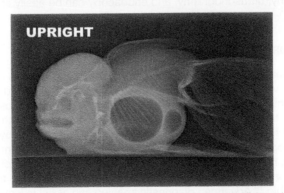

Fig. 7. A horizontal beam right lateral radiograph of a fancy goldfish with buoyancy disorder that was positively buoyant and swimming inverted. Note the cranial chamber of the swim bladder is hyperinflated and can also cause displacement of the caudal chamber. The spine is lordotic and scoliotic; note asymmetric spacing between the dorsal vertebrae. (*Courtesy of* Dr Lori Campbell, University of California at Davis Veterinary Teaching Hospital, Davis, CA.)

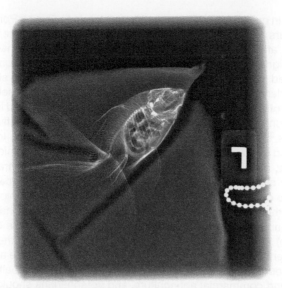

Fig. 8. A left lateral radiograph of a fancy goldfish suffering from buoyancy disorder with severely gas-distended intestines caused by an intestinal pseudo-obstruction. (*Courtesy of* Dr Tracey Ritzman, Davis, CA.)

bladder or gastrointestinal tract, arising from repeated traumatic damage and inflammation to the spinal cord innervation and nerve roots to these organs. Because ideal body conformation of several fancy goldfish varieties result in lordotic and scoliotic spines, damage to nerves and spinal roots can readily occur as a consequence of normal locomotion. Some advanced imaging studies from clinical cases have shown that the spinal canal in affected spines may be reduced by up to 75%. Further studies are needed to identify the normal swim bladder and gastrointestinal innervation in these animals, and research should be complemented with advanced clinical data detailing the consequences of nerve damage to these organs. A variety of palliative treatments to address swim bladder problems have been performed using dietary changes, and several studies of surgical techniques have been published, but all forms of medical and surgical treatments lack a long-lasting or complete curative effect.[31–33] Intestinal pseudo-obstruction in other animals is treated using gastrointestinal motility drugs, and erythromycin may prove to be the most readily available treatment of these fish patients.[34,35]

TOXINS

Because veterinarians are often limited with treatment options, toxins often go undiagnosed or underreported, except in cases of large fish kills. Several environmental toxins can have detrimental effects in fish, and many can subsequently cause human illness if not detected. Many of these ichthyosarcotoxins do not specifically target the gastrointestinal tract in fish, but when ingested in sufficient quantities, many of these agents are neurotoxic and can lead to death. These toxins can include environmental pollutants, heavy metals, and naturally occurring chemicals found in microcystis, cyanobacteria, and dinoflagellates. The most information is available for toxins causing the greatest threat to public health, such as domoic acid and ciguatoxins. Epidemics related to ciguatoxin, produced by the dinoflagellate *Gambierdiscus toxicus* have been associated in cases ranging from the Virgin Islands to French Polynesia.[35] When an outbreak occurs, the most likely reef fish species implicated are the microphagous-grazing fish, and after affected fish are eaten, these toxins cause nausea, vomiting, and neurologic signs in affected persons.[36] In more recent years, domoic acid intoxication has caused greater media attention. Originally identified as a shellfish toxin off Prince Edward Island after a human outbreak associated with mussels,[37] this neurotoxin found in dinoflagellates can accumulate in krill and is implicated in morbidity and mortality events on the Pacific West Coast in brown pelicans, planktivorous fish, and marine mammals.[38–40] After evading diagnosis for several years, a toxin associated with morbidity and mortality in channel catfish was identified as the microcystin *Microcystis aeruginosa*, causing high mortality in commercial catfish operations, although fish showed few clinical signs, affected animals show marked hepatic and splenic congestion and a distended stomach filled with algae containing microcystins found at necropsy.[41] Other mortality events associated with commercial channel catfish epidemics have been associated with ingestion of a toxic form of the blue-green alga (*Cyanobacterium*) *Aphanizomenon flos-aquae*.[42] Although many of these toxic events may not be preventable, it is the responsibility of veterinarians to be aware that these ingested toxins found in fish can have negative effects for public health, wildlife medicine, fisheries, and commercial aquaculture, and veterinarians should also be aware of how to take diagnostic samples associated with mass fish die-offs.

THIAMINE AND TAURINE DEFICIENCY

Appropriate nutrition is critical for the welfare, longevity, performance, and production of aquatic animals. Although the clinical effects and implications of thiamin and taurine deficiency in humans and other mammals are well documented, understanding these requirements for fish is a recent development.

Thiaminase is a naturally occurring endogenous or exogenous enzyme that causes breakdown of the vitamin thiamin, making components inactive for cellular metabolism. Sources of thiaminase include several species of fish from the families Cyprinidae and Clupeidae, fish species commonly used as food sources for other aquatic animals.[43] Thiamine deficiency is a common occurrence for aquatic animals in captivity and wild fisheries, because feeding frozen fish or feeder cyprinid fish is a common practice for predatory fish species, turtles, and aquatic snakes. In captive collections, when juvenile animals are fed fish sources contain thiaminase, thiamine deficiency can have a profound effect on nervous, skeletal, and reproductive development of these fish (**Fig. 9**). Fish fed inappropriate diets develop chronic or nonspecific health problems. The effects of thiaminase can also be observed in aquatic wildlife. Clinical examples of thiamine deficiency were first observed in wild salmonids from the Great Lakes manifesting as lake trout early mortality syndrome,

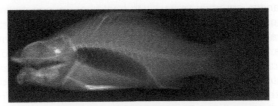

Fig. 9. A right lateral radiograph of a juvenile Nile perch (*Holocentrus adescensionis*) showing skeletal malformations with ventral deviation in dentary and articular bones of the lower jaw associated with thiamine deficiency.

resulting from having normal prey species supplanted by invasive alewifes (*Alosa pseudoharengus*), a fish high in thiaminase.[44] Similarly, thiamin deficiency has been documented for morbid American alligators from Griffin Lake, Florida.[45] These animals showed neurologic signs and pathology consistent with thiamine deficiency, which was proved by further research suggesting the alligators' diet of a high proportion of thiaminase-containing gizzard shad (*Dorosoma cepedianum*) played a role.[46]

Most veterinarians learn about feline taurine deficiency as related to changes associated with commercial cat food diets. There are many clinical signs for taurine deficiency caused by taurine-deficient diets in mammals, but a couple of the most profound findings in domestic cats included retinal degeneration and a reversible.[47,48] Taurine is an essential organic acid needed for various metabolic roles, including bile acid conjugation, membrane stabilization, and calcium signaling.[49] These metabolic functions make taurine necessary for proper cardiac, skeletal muscle, nervous, and retinal development and function.[50] Taurine naturally occurs in seafood and meat, but many vertebrates can synthesize taurine in the pancreas. Some species of animals cannot synthesize taurine and depend on dietary sources. Taurine requirements for fish are just beginning to be understood. Research suggests that many freshwater fish species, including salmonids, are able to synthesize taurine, but many predatory marine species do not have this same pathway.[51] Commercial aquaculture feed producers have been trying to minimize the use of fish protein sources by supplementing with feather meal and soy alternatives in an effort to make more environmentally sensitive choices and to decrease costs.[52,53] Salmonid diets low in taurine may not afford an appropriate dietary formulation that can be equivocally transferred for use in mariculture of marine cobia (*Rachycentron canadum*),[54] red sea bream (*Pagrus major*),[55] *Seriola quinqueradiata*,[56] or *Thunnus* sp. In *Seriola quinqueradiata* and *Pagrus major*, animals developed green liver syndrome and had poor growth performance after being fed a taurine-deficient diet when compared with animals receiving taurine-rich diets.[55,57]

PREBIOTICS AND PROBIOTICS

The gastrointestinal flora of fish is poorly understood, and research generally is restricted to economically important aquaculture species. Some of the early work identifying the gastrointestinal microflora in fish found normal flora to consist mainly of gram-negative rods, with the predominant bacteria comprising *Enterobacter*, *Aeromonas*, and *Acinetobacter* species of freshwater salmonids.[58] In healthy fish, other research showed a greater mixture of gram-negative and gram-positive organisms, with gastrointestinal microbe populations including *Streptococcus*, *Leuconostoc*, *Lactobacillus*, and *Carnobacterium* species.[59] Populations of these lactic acid bacteria in fish were influenced by nutritional and environmental factors like dietary polyunsaturated fatty acids, chromic oxide, stress, and salinity.[59] Comparatively for birds and mammals, gastrointestinal flora has been shown to be affected by prebiotics and probiotics, and in poultry, prebiotics have been identified as having effects on growth, immune function, digestion, disease resistance, and pathogen survival.[60] In vitro, *Lactobacillus bulgaricus* and *Lactobacillus rhamnosus* ATCC 53103, commercially available human-derived and dairy-derived probiotics, were shown to penetrate and adhere to fish mucus, to suppress 3 fish pathogens when grown concomitantly in culture, and to be stable against fish bile.[61] Prebiotics and probiotics may treat and prevent infectious diseases, could enhance oral medication and vaccine uptake, and can better maintain healthy and normal gastrointestinal flora in fish.[62] More

Table 1
Piscine gastrointestinal differential diagnosis. Select fish pathogens including the World Organization for Animal Health (OIE) and US Department of Agriculture (USDA) reportable diseases listing the cause, species, and gastrointestinal-related clinical signs, and including select primary zoonotic bacterial pathogens of fish listing associated human clinical signs caused by these pathogens

	Cause	Species	Associated Gastrointestinal Signs (Nonspecific)
OIE and USDA[65,66]	Epizootic hematopoietic necrosis virus (EHNV): Iridoviridae[67]	Redfin perch, rainbow trout, families Salmonidae and Percidae	Swollen coelom and abdominal ascites
Reportable diseases	Epizootic ulcerative syndrome (EUS): oomycete Aphanomyces invadans or A piscicida[68]	Ornamental tropicals and warm water foodfish, nonspecific	Loss of appetite
	Gyrodactylosis (Gyrodactylus salaris): monogenean ectoparasite[69]	Atlantic salmon (Salmo salar)	Loss of appetite
	Infectious hematopoietic necrosis virus (IHNV): Rhabdoviridae[70]	Family Salmonidae	Coelomic distension, long, semitransparent fecal casts often trail from the anus
	Infectious salmon anemia virus (ISAV): Orthomyxoviridae[71]	Atlantic salmon (Salmo salar) but some Pacific salmonids can carry virus without clinical signs	Loss of appetite
	Koi herpesvirus disease (CyHV3): Herpesviridae[72]	Some members of family Cyprinidae, including Cyprinus carpio	Anorexia, severe wasting
	Red sea bream iridoviral disease (RSIVD): Iridoviridae[73]	A variety of marine temperate and warm water species, nonspecific	Coelomic distension and ascites, loss of appetite
	Spring viremia of carp virus (SVCV): Rhabdoviridae[74]	Carp and other fish in family Cyprinidae	Coelomic distension, inflammation or edema of the vent (often with trailing mucoid fecal casts)
	Viral hemorrhagic septicemia virus (VHSV): Rhabdoviridae[75]	A variety of freshwater and marine temperate species	Coelomic distension and ascites, loss of appetite
Bacterial zoonotic pathogens of fish	Aeromonas spp: bacteria[76,77]	A variety of fresh water animals in cold to warm water environments	In fish, most commonly associated with dermal lesions, but intestinal enterocytes also infected; human contamination from infected water causes necrotizing skin lesions or acute gastroenteritis

Edwardsiella tarda: bacteria[78,79]	Marine and freshwater species of fish including salmonids, channel catfish (*Ictalurus* sp), eels (*Anguilla* sp)	Coelomic swelling, rectal hernia, hemorrhagic ascites enlarged and congested liver; in humans this manifests as enteric disease
Enteric redmouth disease (*Yersinia ruckeri*): bacteria[80]	Salmonids susceptible but nonspecific	Reddening of throat and mouth in fish, anorexia; humans severe gastroenteritis
Atypical mycobacteriosis – *Mycobacterium* ssp (*chelonae, fortuitum, marinum,* and so forth)[81-84]	Nonspecific infections of temperate and warm water fishes	Lethargy, coelomic distension, ascites, anorexia, severe wasting with voracious appetite, external ulcers, gray-white granulomas anywhere on body or internal organs especially liver, kidney, and spleen; human infections are marked by nonhealing wounds, generally on distal ends of extremities that may involve bony tissues
Salmonella spp[85,86]	Nonspecific, warm water ornamental and food fish	Fish have no clinical signs; humans show abdominal pain, acute gastroenteritis, bloody mucoid diarrhea, nausea, vomiting, fever
Streptococcus inaie[87]	Warm water aquaculture *Tilapia* sp, nonspecific	Coelomic distension and ascites; humans usually cellulitis unless immunocompromised
Piscine pasteurellosis: *Photobacterium damsela* ssp *Piscicida*[88]	Nonspecific, a variety of warm water and temperate marine fishes	Coelomic distension and ascites marked by hemorrhagic septicemia, granulomas in the spleen, kidney and liver; humans causes necrotizing fasciitis
Family Vibrionaceae: *Plesiomonas shigelloides*[89-92]	Nonspecific in both fish and shellfish, ubiquitous pathogens in water environment	Shellfish nonclinical, fish most commonly have clinical signs associated with hemorrhagic disease and skin lesion but some *Vibrio* sp can cause gastroenteritis; humans have diarrhea, nausea, vomiting, fever, chills, and abdominal pain

research is needed to better understand the role of prebiotics and probiotics on piscine gastrointestinal physiology.

INFECTIOUS AGENTS

Infectious agents from viruses to parasitic clams can cause disease in fish, leading to varying levels of morbidity and mortality. Historically, fish health has focused on parasitic infections, although advances in molecular biology have broadened our knowledge regarding microbial pathogens in the last 3 decades. These improvements in research methodology and equipment for human and small animal veterinary medicine are helping to further our understanding of the pathogenesis of infectious diseases in aquatic animal health. Traditionally, few fish pathogens had been associated as zoonotic diseases, but because of improved laboratory technologies, some of these pathogens are being implicated as human pathogens and are of significant concern. Aeromonads, common pathogens associated with skin ulceration and erosions of salmonids and cyprinids, are being associated with enteritis in humans.[63] This finding suggests that a similar syndrome may persist in fish chronically infected with *Aeromonas* sp that show signs of gastroenteritis. To show how new laboratory tools can advance fish health research, *Edwardsiella tarda*, another zoonotic fish pathogen, was investigated using green fluorescent protein-tagged bacteria to investigate the portal of entry for this pathogen in vivo.[64] Ling and colleagues[64] identified the gastrointestinal tract as a port of entry in the blue gourami, *Trichogaster trichopterus*, suggesting that the colonization of the intestines by this pathogen may overcome gastric acid secretions similar to mechanisms occurring with other more commonly known food-borne pathogens. Some common examples of reportable and zoonotic fish diseases and syndromic gastrointestinal signs are summarized in **Table 1**.

SUMMARY

Veterinary gastroenterology in fish continues to be a growing area for new research and clinical treatments. Advanced diagnostic techniques can be practically modified and directly applied to fish patients for identifying gastrointestinal ailments. There may be a greater role for probiotics and prebiotics in aquaculture nutrition. More research investigating the normal intestinal flora of fish, the oral pharmacokinetics for both drugs and vaccines, the optimal nutritional requirements for various species, and the role of mucosal immunity on protection against common fish pathogens serves to improve our veterinary approach for a broader and more comprehensive understanding of fish gastroenterology.

ACKNOWLEDGMENTS

I dedicate this article to Dr Rocco Cipriano, a scientist studying fish health for more than 30 years with the US Geological Survey at the National Fish Health Research Laboratory in Leetown, WV.

Rocco also began building collaborations among fisheries biologists, coral disease researchers, laboratory diagnosticians, and veterinarians working in aquatic animal health through his tireless efforts to organize, coordinate, and run the Eastern Fish Health Workshop (EFHW) over the last 20+ years. During these meetings, Rocco stresses sound science, but he also constantly evolves the EFHW programmatically to include new and emerging issues, incorporate veterinary continuing education, and provide a welcoming atmosphere for professional mentoring, especially for new participants and students. As an extension of the EFHW, Rocco also fostered sharing aquatic animal health internationally with three Russian/US bilateral conferences, emphasizing the same successful principles used to execute the EFHW every year. The clinical case included in this article was presented at the third US-Russia Conference on Aquatic Animal Health on July 13–17, 2009 in Shepherdstown, WV.

REFERENCES

1. Weber ES. Gastroenterology for the piscine patient. Veterinary Clin North Am Exot Anim Pract 2005;8(2):247–76.
2. Eschmeyer WN, editor. Catalog of fishes. California Academy of Sciences Available at: http://research.calacademy.org/research/ichthyology/catalog/fishcatmain.asp. Accessed February 3, 2013.
3. Fricke R, editor. Catalog of fishes. Literature. Available at: http://research.cal academy.org/research/ichthyology/catalog/fishcatmain.asp. Accessed February 2, 2013.
4. Eschmeyer WN, Fricke R, Fong JD, et al. Marine fish diversity: history of knowledge and discovery (Pisces). Zootaxa 2010;2525:19–50.
5. Blake IH. Studies on the comparative histology of the digestive tube of certain teleost fishes. III. A bottom-feeding fish, the sea robin (Prionotus carolinus). J Morphol 1936;60(1):77–102.
6. Owen R. On the anatomy of vertebrates: fishes and reptiles (Vol. 1). Longman, Green, 1866.
7. Wolf JC, Wolfe MJ. A brief overview of nonncoplastic hepatic toxicity in fish. Toxicol Pathol 2005;33(1):75–85.
8. Blake IH. Studies on the comparative histology of the digestive tube of certain teleost fishes. I. A predaceous fish, the sea bass (Centropristes striatus). J Morphol 1930;50(1):39–70.
9. Rogick MD. Studies on the comparative histology of the digestive tube of certain teleost fishes II. A minnow (Campostoma anomalum). J Morphol 1931;52(1):1–25.
10. Greene CW. Anatomy and histology of the alimentary tract of the king salmon. Government Printing Office. 1913; 777.
11. Chakrabarti I, Gani MA, Chaki KK, et al. Digestive enzymes in 11 freshwater teleost fish species in relation to food habit and niche segregation. Comp Biochem Physiol Physiol 1955;112(1):167–77.
12. Zambonino Infante JL, Cahu CL. Ontogeny of the gastrointestinal tract of marine fish larvae. Comp Biochem Physiol C Toxicol Pharmacol 2001;130(4):477–87.
13. Hart S, Wrathmell AB, Harris JE, et al. Gut immunology in fish: a review. Dev Comp Immunol 1988;12(3):453–80.
14. McMillan DN, Secombes CJ. Isolation of rainbow trout (Oncorhynchus mykiss) intestinal intraepithelial lymphocytes (IEL) and measurement of their cytotoxic activity. Fish & Shellfish Immunology 1997;7(8):527–41.
15. McLean E, Donaldson EM. Absorption of bioactive proteins by the gastrointestinal tract of fish: a review. J Aquat Anim Health 1980;2(1):1–11.
16. Weber EP, Weisse C, Schwarz T, et al. Anesthesia, diagnostic imaging, and surgery of fish. Compend Contin Educ Vet 2009;2:E1–9.
17. Hernandez-Divers SJ, Bakal RS, Hickson BH, et al. Endoscopic sex determination and gonadal manipulation in Gulf of Mexico sturgeon (Acipenser oxyrinchus desotoi). J Zoo Wildl Med 2004;35(4):459–70.
18. Swenson EA, Rosenberger AE, Howell PJ. Validation of endoscopy for determination of maturity in small salmonids and sex of mature individuals. Trans Am Fish Soc 2007;136(4):994–8.

19. Wildgoose WH. Internal diseases of ornamental fish: a clinical approach. 2006; Bulletin - European Association of Fish Pathologists, 26(1), 46.
20. Beregi A, Szekely CS, Békési L. Radiodiagnostic examination of the swimbladder of some fish species. Acta Vet Hung 2001;49(1):87–98.
21. Pees M, Pees K, Kiefer I. The use of computed tomography for assessment of the swim bladder in Koi Carp (Cyprinus carpio). Vet Radiol Ultrasound 2010; 51(3):294–8.
22. Trouillier A, El-Matbouli M, Hoffmann RW. A new look at the life-cycle of Hoferellus carassii in the goldfish (Carassius auratus auratus) and its relation to "kidney enlargement disease" (KED). Folia Parasitol 1996;43(3):173–87.
23. Weisse C, Weber ES, Matzkin Z, et al. Surgical removal of a seminoma from a black sea bass. J Am Vet Med Assoc 2002;221(2):280–3.
24. Lewbart GA, Spodnick G, Barlow N, et al. Surgical removal of an undifferentiated abdominal sarcoma from a koi carp (Cyprinus carpio). Vet Rec 1998; 143(20):556–8.
25. Harms CA, Bakal RS, Khoo LH, et al. Microsurgical excision of an abdominal mass in a gourami. J Am Vet Med Assoc 1995;207(9):1215.
26. Kapur RP. Neuropathology of paediatric chronic intestinal pseudo-obstruction and related animal models. J Pathol 2001;194(3):277–88.
27. Sullivan MA, Snape WJ Jr, Matarazzo SA, et al. Gastrointestinal myoelectrical activity in idiopathic intestinal pseudo-obstruction. N Engl J Med 1977;297(5): 233–8.
28. Stanghellini V, Camilleri M, Malagelada JR. Chronic idiopathic intestinal pseudo-obstruction: clinical and intestinal manometric findings. Gut 1987;28(1):5–12.
29. Arbuatti A, Della Salda L, Romanucci M. Pathology survey on a captive-bred colony of the Mexican Goodeid, nearly extinct in the wild, Zoogoneticus tequila (Webb & Miller 1998). ScientificWorldJournal 2013;2013:401468.
30. Grizzle JM, Curd MR. Posthatching histological development of the digestive system and swim bladder of logperch, Percina caprodes. Copeia 1978;448–55.
31. Lewbart GA, Stone EA, Love NE. Pneumocystectomy in a Midas cichlid. J Am Vet Med Assoc 1995;207(3):319–21.
32. Britt T, Weisse C, Weber ES, et al. Use of pneumocystoplasty for overinflation of the swim bladder in a goldfish. J Am Vet Med Assoc 2002;221(5):690–3.
33. Lewbart GA, Christian LS, Dombrowski D. Development of a minimally invasive technique to stabilize buoyancy-challenged goldfish (Carassius auratus). Presented at the 36th annual International Association for Aquatic Animal Medicine. The Alaska SeaLife Center and Alaskan IAAAM Seward, Alaska, May 14–18, 2005.
34. Emmanuel AV, Shand AG, Kamm MA. Erythromycin for the treatment of chronic intestinal pseudo-obstruction: description of six cases with a positive response. Aliment Pharmacol Ther 2004;19(6):687–94.
35. Weber FH Jr, Richards RD, McCallum RW. Erythromycin: a motilin agonist and gastrointestinal prokinetic agent. Am J Gastroenterol 1993;88(4):485–90.
36. Engleberg NC, Morris JG, Lewis J, et al. Ciguatera fish poisoning: a major common-source outbreak in the US Virgin Islands. Ann Intern Med 1983; 98(3):336–7.
37. Bagnis R, Chanteau S, Chungue E, et al. Origins of ciguatera fish poisoning: a new dinoflagellate, Gambierdiscus toxicus Adachi and Fukuyo, definitively involved as a causal agent. Toxicon 1980;18(2):199–208.
38. Bates SS, Bird CJ, Freitas AD, et al. Pennate diatom Nitzschia pungens as the primary source of domoic acid, a toxin in shellfish from eastern Prince Edward Island, Canada. Can Tech Rep Fish Aquat Sci 1989;46(7):1203–15.

39. Work TM, Barr B, Beale AM, et al. Epidemiology of domoic acid poisoning in brown pelicans (*Pelecanus occidentalis*) and Brandt's cormorants (*Phalacrocorax penicillatus*) in California. J Zoo Wildl Med 1993;54–62.

40. Lefebvre K, Silver M, Coale S, et al. Domoic acid in planktivorous fish in relation to toxic *Pseudonitzschia* cell densities. Mar Biol 2002;140(3):625–31.

41. Lefebvre KA, Powell CL, Busman M, et al. Detection of domoic acid in northern anchovies and California sea lions associated with an unusual mortality event. Nat Toxins 1999;7(3):85–92.

42. Zimba PV, Khoo L, Gaunt PS, et al. Confirmation of catfish, *Ictalurus punctatus* (Rafinesque), mortality from *Microcystis* toxins. J Fish Dis 2001;24(1):41–7.

43. Nonneman D, Zimba PV. A PCR-based test to assess the potential for microcystin occurrence in channel catfish production ponds. J Phycol 2002;38(1):230–3.

44. Wistbacka S, Lönnström LG, Bonsdorff E, et al. Thiaminase activity of crucian carp *Carassius carassius* injected with a bacterial fish pathogen, *Aeromonas salmonicida* subsp. salmonicida. J Aquat Anim Health 2009;21(4):217–28.

45. Brown SB, Fitzsimons JD, Palace VP, et al. Thiamine and early mortality syndrome in lake trout. In Early life stage mortality syndrome in fishes of the Great Lakes and Baltic Sea. American Fisheries Society, Symposium 21. Dearborn (MI): American Fisheries Society; 1996. p. 18–25.

46. Schoeb TR, Heaton-Jones TG, Clemmons RM, et al. Clinical and necropsy findings associated with increased mortality among American alligators of Lake Griffin, Florida. J Wildl Dis 2002;38(2):320–37.

47. Honeyfield DC, Ross JP, Carbonneau DA, et al. Pathology, physiologic parameters, tissue contaminants, and tissue thiamine in morbid and healthy central Florida adult American alligators (*Alligator mississippiensis*). J Wildl Dis 2008; 44(2):280–94.

48. Hayes KC, Carey RE, Schmidt SY. Retinal degeneration associated with taurine deficiency in the cat. Science 1975;188(4191):949–51.

49. Pion PD, Kittleson MD, Rogers QR, et al. Myocardial failure in cats associated with low plasma taurine: a reversible cardiomyopathy. Science 1987; 237(4816):764–8.

50. Huxtable RJ. Physiological actions of taurine. Physiol Rev 1992;72(1):101–63.

51. Yokoyama M, Takeuchi T, Park GS, et al. Hepatic cysteinesulphinate decarboxylase activity in fish. Aquaculture Res 2001;32(s1):216–20.

52. Li P, Mai K, Trushenski J, et al. New developments in fish amino acid nutrition: towards functional and environmentally oriented aquafeeds. Amino Acids 2009;37(1):43–53.

53. Jirsa D, Davis A, Stuart K, et al. Development of a practical soy-based diet for California yellowtail, *Seriola lalandi*. Aquaculture Nutr 2011;17(4):e869–74.

54. Lunger AN, McLean E, Gaylord TG, et al. Taurine supplementation to alternative dietary proteins used in fish meal replacement enhances growth of juvenile cobia (*Rachycentron canadum*). Aquaculture 2007;271(1):401–10.

55. Takagi S, Murata H, Goto T, et al. Efficacy of taurine supplementation for preventing green liver syndrome and improving growth performance in yearling red sea bream *Pagrus major* fed low-fishmeal diet. Rev Fish Sci 2006;72(6):1191–9.

56. Takagi S, Murata H, Goto T, et al. Taurine is an essential nutrient for yellowtail *Seriola quinqueradiata* fed non-fish meal diets based on soy protein concentrate. Aquaculture 2008;280(1):198–205.

57. Takagi S, Murata H, Goto T, et al. The green liver syndrome is caused by taurine deficiency in yellowtail, *Seriola quinqueradiata* fed diets without fishmeal. Suisan Zoshoku 2005;53(3):279.

58. Trust TJ, Sparrow RA. The bacterial flora in the alimentary tract of freshwater salmonid fishes. Can J Microbiol 1974;20(9):1219–28.
59. Ringø E, Gatesoupe FJ. Lactic acid bacteria in fish: a review. Aquaculture 1998; 160(3):177–203.
60. Patterson JA, Burkholder KM. Application of prebiotics and probiotics in poultry production. Poult Sci 2003;82(4):627–31.
61. Nikoskelainen S, Salminen S, Bylund G, et al. Characterization of the properties of human-and dairy-derived probiotics for prevention of infectious diseases in fish. Appl Environ Microbiol 2001;67(6):2430–5.
62. Burr G, Gatlin D, Ricke S. Microbial ecology of the gastrointestinal tract of fish and the potential application of prebiotics and probiotics in finfish aquaculture. J World Aquaculture Soc 2005;36(4):425–36.
63. Janda JM, Abbott SL. Evolving concepts regarding the genus *Aeromonas*: an expanding panorama of species, disease presentations, and unanswered questions. Clin Infect Dis 1998;27(2):332–44.
64. Ling SH, Wang XH, Lim TM, et al. Green fluorescent protein-tagged *Edwardsiella tarda* reveals portal of entry in fish. FEMS Microbiol Lett 2001;194(2):239–43.
65. Available at: http://www.aphis.usda.gov/animal_health/animal_dis_spec/aqua culture/. Accessed October 1, 2013.
66. Available at: http://www.oie.int/international-standard-setting/aquatic-code/ access-online/. Accessed October 1, 2013.
67. Langdon JS, Humphrey JD, Williams LM. Outbreaks of an EHNV-like iridovirus in cultured rainbow trout, *Salmo gairdneri* Richardson, in Australia. J Fish Dis 1988; 11(1):93–6.
68. Egusa S, Masuda N. A new fungal disease of *Plecoglossus altivelis*. Fish Pathol 1971;6:41–6.
69. Bakke TA, Jansen PA, Hansen LP. Differences in the host resistance of Atlantic salmon, *Salmo salar* L. stocks to the monogenean *Gyrodactylus salaris* Malmberg. J Fish Biol 1957;1990(37):577–87.
70. Fish diseases. In: Schäperclaus W, Kulow H, Schreckenbach K, editors. Infectious hematopoietic necrosis (IHN). 5th editon. Rotterdam (The Netherlands): AA Balkema; 1992. p. 345–9.
71. Raynard RS, Murray AG, Gregory A. Infectious salmon anaemia virus in wild fish from Scotland. Dis Aquat Org 2001;46(2):93–100.
72. Hedrick RP, Gilad O, Yun S, et al. A herpesvirus associated with mass mortality of juvenile and adult koi, a strain of common carp. J Aquat Anim Health 2000; 12(1):44–57.
73. Inouye K, Yamano K, Maeno Y, et al. Iridovirus infection of cultured red sea bream, *Pagrus major*. Fish Pathol 1992;27:19–27.
74. Goodwin AE. First report of spring viremia of carp virus (SVCV) in North America. J Aquat Anim Health 2002;14(3):161–4.
75. Winton JR, Batts WN, Nishizawa T, et al. Characterization of the first North American isolates of viral hemorrhagic septicemia virus. Fish Health Sect Am Fish Soc 1989;17(2):2.
76. Ringø E, Jutfelt F, Kanapathippillai P, et al. Damaging effect of the fish pathogen *Aeromonas salmonicida* ssp. *salmonicida* on intestinal enterocytes of Atlantic salmon (*Salmo salar* L.). Cell Tissue Res 2004;318(2):305–11.
77. Boulanger Y, Lallier R, Cousineau G. Isolation of enterotoxigenic *Aeromonas* from fish. Can J Microbiol 1977;23(9):1161–4.
78. Berg RW, Anderson AW. *Salmonellae* and *Edwardsiella tarda* in gull feces: a source of contamination in fish processing plants. Appl Microbiol 1972;24(3):501–3.

79. Park SB, Aoki T, Jung TS. Pathogenesis of and strategies for preventing *Edwardsiella tarda* infection in fish. Vet Res 2012;43(1):1–11.
80. Furones MD, Rodgers CJ, Munn CB. *Yersinia ruckeri*, the causal agent of enteric redmouth disease (ERM) in fish. Annu Rev Fish Dis 1993;3:105–25.
81. Beran V, Matlova L, Dvorska L, et al. Distribution of mycobacteria in clinically healthy ornamental fish and their aquarium environment. J Fish Dis 2006; 29(7):383–93.
82. Decostere A, Hermans K, Haesebrouck F. Piscine mycobacteriosis: a literature review covering the agent and the disease it causes in fish and humans. Vet Microbiol 2004;99(3):159–66.
83. Dulin MP. A review of tuberculosis (mycobacteriosis) in fish. Vet Med Small Anim Clin 1979;74(5):731.
84. Jacobs JM, Stine CB, Baya AM, et al. A review of mycobacteriosis in marine fish. J Fish Dis 2009;32(2):119–30.
85. Heinitz ML, Ruble RD, Wagner DE, et al. Incidence of *Salmonella* in fish and sea-food. J Food Prot 2000;63(5):579–92.
86. Musto J, Kirk M, Lightfoot D, et al. Multi-drug resistant *Salmonella Java* infections acquired from tropical fish aquariums, Australia 2003–04. Commun Dis Intell 2006;30(2):222.
87. Weinstein MR, Litt M, Kertesz DA, et al. Invasive infections due to a fish pathogen, *Streptococcus iniae*. N Engl J Med 1997;337(9):589–94.
88. Zorrilla I, Balebona MC, Sarasquete C, et al. Isolation and characterization of the causative agent of pasteurellosis, *Photobacterium damsela* ssp *piscicida*, from sole, *Solea senegalensis* (Kaup) J Fish Dis 1999;22(3):167–72.
89. Kain KC, Kelly MT. Clinical features, epidemiology, and treatment of *Plesiomonas shigelloides* diarrhea. J Clin Microbiol 1989;27(5):998–1001.
90. Munn CB. Vibriosis in fish and its control. Aquaculture Res 1977;8(1):11–5.
91. Egidius E. Vibriosis: pathogenicity and pathology. A review. Aquaculture 1987; 67(1):15–28.
92. Colwell RR, Grimes DJ. Vibrio diseases of marine fish populations. Helgoländer Meeresuntersuchungen 1984;37(1–4):265–87.

Pathology of the Exotic Companion Mammal Gastrointestinal System

Drury Reavill, DVM, DABVP (Avian and Reptile & Amphibian Practice), DACVP

KEYWORDS

- Chinchilla • Gerbil • Hamster • Mouse • Rabbit • Rat • Sugar glider
- Gastrointestinal disease

KEY POINTS

- A variety of disease agents can affect the gastrointestinal tract, some of which can pose zoonotic health concerns.
- Many conditions are present with nonspecific clinical signs (lethargy, variable degrees of diarrhea, and for most sick rodents, presenting hunched with spiky fur), necessitating additional laboratory testing to reach a diagnosis.
- Primary tumors of the digestive tract are also presented as well as miscellaneous conditions ranging from toxins to trauma.

INTRODUCTION

This review covers gastrointestinal and select oral diseases from rodent submissions to the author's laboratory[1] as well as some classic diseases from the literature. There is limited information on clinical sign presentations and potential therapies. The disease agents cover viruses, bacteria, fungi, protozoans, and metazoan parasites. Primary tumors of the digestive tract are described as well as miscellaneous conditions ranging from toxins to trauma.

CHINCHILLA
Oral Disease

Chinchillas have continuously growing open-rooted (hypsodontic) teeth. Malocclusion of these teeth can involve the incisors, premolars, and molars. Overgrowth and abnormal wear may result in sharp points and edges to the teeth as well as fractures of the tooth. These sharp edges traumatize the oral cavity, leading to gingivitis, stomatitis, and glossitis. The common presentation of dental disease is lethargy, anorexia,

Disclosure: This article originally appeared in similar form in the proceedings of the 2013 Association of Exotic Mammal Veterinarians Conference in Indianapolis, Indiana, USA.
Zoo/Exotic Pathology Service, 2825 KOVR Drive, West Sacramento, CA 95605, USA
E-mail address: Dreavill@zooexotic.com

Vet Clin Exot Anim 17 (2014) 145–164
http://dx.doi.org/10.1016/j.cvex.2014.01.002
1094-9194/14/$ – see front matter © 2014 Elsevier Inc. All rights reserved.

and hypersalivation.[2] Radiographic studies have proved to be a valuable tool to completely evaluate malocclusion.[3] The cause(s) may be familial or the result of trauma or inappropriate dietary items or infections.

Gastrointestinal Tract

Bacteria

A variety of bacteria are reported to cause enteritis. Published reports describe *Klebsiella pneumoniae*,[4] *Yersinia enterocolitica* (classically producing a fibrinous enterocolitis),[5] *Listeria monocytogenes*,[6] *Staphylococcus*,[7] *Pseudomonas aeruginosa*, and *Proteus mirabilis*[8] as agents of disease.

Gastroenteritis caused by *Klebsiella pneumoniae* also resulted in an acute systemic infection in a chinchilla breeding colony.[4] The author has found that *Klebsiella pneumoniae* remains a common cause of enteritis and systemic infections in young chinchillas.

Yersinia enterocolitica has been associated with sporadic outbreaks of deaths in chinchilla colonies. The lesions were of granulomatous hepatitis, splenitis, and fibrinous enterocolitis, closely resembling the classic lesions of *Yersinia pseudotuberculosis*.[5]

Listeria monocytogenes is an obligate intracellular bacterium that causes 3 distinct clinical entities: septicemia, encephalitis, and abortion. The septicemic form affects the viscera with or without meningoencephalitis and is common in monogastric animals, whereas encephalitis and abortion occur principally in adult ruminants. Historically, chinchillas are considered one of the species more susceptible to visceral listeriosis, especially when reared in confinement. The lesions include emaciation, multiple white foci on the capsular/serosal surfaces and parenchyma of the liver, mesenteric lymph nodes, and intestines, including the cecum and colon. Rectal prolapses and colonic intussusception also occurred (**Fig. 1**).[9] These lesions grossly resemble infections by *Salmonella* sp as well as *Yersinia pseudotuberculosis*. Histologically, the intestines have transmural inflammation effacing the Peyer patches of the small intestine and multifocal inflammation of cecum and colon.[6] The source of infection is usually from foodstuffs.[9] *Listeria ivanovii*, a more common isolate from cattle and sheep, has also been identified in chinchillas, resulting in septicemia. The intestines were noted to have mucoid contents.[10]

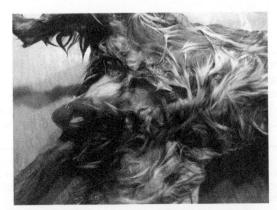

Fig. 1. Rectal prolapse in a chinchilla. Bacterial enteritis, enteropathy caused by *Clostridium perfringens* type A enterotoxin, and severe pinworm infections are associated with prolapses in rodents.

Staphylococcal enterocolitis is a complication of antibiotic therapy, particularly broad-spectrum antibiotics, in chinchillas.[7] The bacterial overgrowth results in a fatal diarrhea and lesion of an ulcerative pseudomembranous enterocolitis.

A *Pseudomonas aeruginosa* and *Proteus mirabilis* disease outbreak resulted in gastritis with a grossly noted excessive mucus accumulating in the lumen as well as an enteritis.[8] It was thought that these animals may have been exposed to contaminated water as the source of the infection.

Protozoa

Cryptosporidia is associated with severe diarrhea in young chinchillas.[11] The small spherical protozoa can be found on the epithelial surface of the stomach, small intestine, and colon. Mucosal villus atrophy is noted with the infection.

It is reported that chinchillas normally have low numbers of intestinal *Giardia*, and the prevalence in pet populations can be significant (30%–66%).[12–14] Age, stress, and poor husbandry are responsible for proliferation of the protozoa and the development of diarrhea. From a survey by the author, most cases were of young animals (6–12 months) and most had other more significant lesions responsible for death.[1] The parasite, *Giardia duodenalis*, should be considered a zoonotic threat, although this issue is unresolved. The organisms are piriform, flattened, 5 to 6 μm long lining the brush border of the villi in the small intestine, duodenum, and cranial jejunum (**Fig. 2**). Transmission is fecal-oral.

Metazoan

The literature has few reports on metazoan enteropathics in chinchillas. Rarely, cases of *Hymenolepis nana* var fraterna are described. The clinical signs are nonspecific, with weight loss and terminal diarrhea. The cestodes reside in the small intestine. One associated lesion was an intussusception.[15] The life cycle of this cestode is unique; infections can occur by direct ingestion of the eggs, or by eating grain beetles infected with cysticercoids, or by autoinfection.

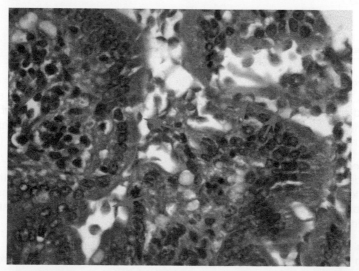

Fig. 2. *Giardia* protozoa are indicated by the red arrows. *Giardia* infections are more commonly described in chinchillas, hamsters, mice, and sugar glider (hematoxylin-eosin, original magnification ×400).

Miscellaneous

Outbreaks of unexpected death in colonies of chinchillas with gastrointestinal clinical signs (diarrhea, rectal prolapses) have been caused by *Clostridium perfringens* type A enterotoxin. Mortality was high. The predominant findings at postmortem were inflammation of the gastrointestinal tract, hepatomegaly, and splenomegly. Microscopic changes consisted of centrilobular necrosis of the liver, edema, congestion and necrosis of the large intestine mucosal, and proliferation of the white pulp of the spleen. The toxin was detected in gastric contents.[16]

Clostridium perfringens (type D) toxin generally results in unexpected death in young chinchillas (2–4 months).[17]

Some cases of typhlitis have a history of cecal stasis. Abrupt diet change, stress, low-fiber diet, and inappropriate antibiotic use have been reported as causes.

Intestinal strictures and intussusceptions are also described, without identifying a definitive cause.[1]

Neoplasia

Of the rare tumors reported in chinchillas,[18] 1 poorly differentiated carcinoma of the salivary gland[19] and an infiltrative gastric adenocarcinoma are described.[20]

The salivary gland tumor presented as a slow-growing, soft, nonpainful mass on the ventral neck. This older chinchilla (12 years) was euthanized 8 months after the mass was identified. The large tumor supported a pleomorphic cellular pattern with pseudocysts. Metastases were present in the submandibular lymph node, liver, lungs, and spleen.[19]

A 5-year-old female chinchilla died after a short period of lethargy and anorexia. On gross examination, the gastric wall was markedly thickened and the lumen almost completely filled with a firm, white, transmural mass. The tumor mass was an infiltrative adenocarcinoma and was not identified in other tissues. Polymerase chain reaction for *Helicobacter pylori* on a section of the stomach was positive; however; this bacterium was not found by silver stains or immunohistochemistry. *H pylori* has been associated with gastric adenocarcinomas in hamsters[21] and induced in gerbils.[20,22]

GERBIL
Gastrointestinal Tract

Bacteria

Gerbils are reported to be very susceptible to *Clostridium piliforme* (Tyzzer disease) infections. These young animals, less than 3 months of age, present with an acute onset of dyspnea, dehydration, and lethargy. Most animals have a triad of lesions, with enteritis/colitis, hepatitis, and myocarditis. The lesions include multifocal hepatic necrosis, necrotizing ileotyphlitis, and colitis with focal myocardial necrosis (**Fig. 3**).

Miscellaneous

Stress-induced gastric ulcers are generally found in the glandular portion of the stomach. The lesion is also seen in rats, hamsters, and guinea pigs.[23] The stressors can include abrupt changes in dietary items, overcrowding, poor housing sanitation, and transporting the animals.

Neoplasia

Tumors in gerbils are uncommonly reported. A squamous cell carcinoma arose from the gingival in 1 gerbil. No metastases were found.[24]

Two adenocarcinomas and 1 cystadenocarcinoma were identified in the cecum of gerbils older than 1 year. The tumors all filled the lumen of the cecum with invasion to

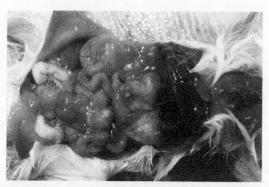

Fig. 3. The liver is swollen with rounded edges and irregular brown areas of hepatic necrosis (*red arrow*). The intestines are gas filled in this gerbil (*red arrowheads*).

the outer muscular wall.[25] One of the cases had a metastasis to the liver.[26] An adenocarcinoma of the stomach also metastasized.[24]

Systemic mastocytosis developed in a 10-month-old female. Although many organs systems were involved, the gastrointestinal tract mucosa was thickened with the proliferating mast cells. The gerbil presented emaciated and with diarrhea.[27]

GUINEA PIG
Oral Disease

Malocclusion results when the continuously growing, open-rooted teeth are not aligned and therefore do not wear properly. Premolars and molars are most often affected. Nutritional or toxic factors (eg, fluorosis) have been incriminated, but it is considered by most to be an inherited condition. As with chinchillas, the points and sharp edges can traumatize the soft tissue of the oral cavity. Severe overgrowth can even trap the tongue (**Fig. 4**). Guinea pigs are at increased risk of tongue entrapment, because of the more acute normal angle of their cheek teeth compared with other exotic mammal species.

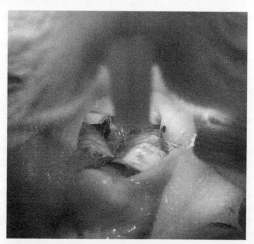

Fig. 4. Malocclusion of the molars has entrapped the tongue of this guinea pig. (*Courtesy of* Teresa Lightfoot, DVM, Tampa, FL.)

Gastrointestinal Tract

Bacteria

Salmonellosis is probably the most important disease of guinea pigs maintained in colonies. It is uncommon in the pet population. Many serotypes may be involved, but usually it is *Salmonella typhimurium* or *Salmonella enteritidis*. The portal of entry is generally by ingestion of food or water contaminated by excreta from wild rodents and birds and rarely through the conjunctiva. *Salmonella* infections can range from latent to acute, subacute, or chronic infections. Latent infections can become overt with stress. Acute infections are generally systemic. Chronic infections are the most common, and by the time they are diagnosed, they can be well established in a colony. Morbidity may approach 100%, and recovered animals may become carriers. Clinical signs are often nonspecific, and diarrhea is uncommon. In chronic disease, there are disseminated pyogranulomas.[28]

Protozoa

Eimeria caviae is identified as an infection of young animals. There is moderate morbidity and mortality. The large intestine and cecum are generally dilated, with dark green to brown fluid feces. In severe infections, the colonic wall is hyperemic, and the mucosa has petechial hemorrhages. Microscopically, there are many developmental stages causing necrosis in the epithelium. In clinically affected guinea pigs, diarrhea, dehydration, weight loss, and death may occur. *E caviae* has a typical eimerian life cycle. Sporulation takes 2 to 11 days, with an average under most conditions of 5 days, so frequent cleaning can prevent reinfection.

Cryptosporidium wrairi may result in death in young guinea pigs. There is poor weight gain and, uncommonly, diarrhea. The organisms can be identified in the small intestine; they are very small, round to oval, and are embedded in the brush border. Infected villi are shortened, broadened, and sometimes flattened. Mild inflammation is occasionally present.

Miscellaneous

Use of some antibiotics that have activity against gram-positive bacteria can suppress normal flora and permit overgrowth of anaerobic and gram-negative bacteria. Toxins produced by 1 anaerobe, *Clostridium difficile*, can result in diarrhea, depression, and death. The intestines are distended with gas and fluid.

Imperforate anus results from failure of anal membranes to perforate, which normally occurs during the first trimester. This condition is not always externally evident in newborn guinea pigs. These animals do not survive long. Intussusceptions are common concurrent lesions.

Dilation or torsion of the stomach or cecum is not uncommon (**Fig. 5**). These guinea pigs are generally found dead, with no clinical signs. An underlying cause is not always determined.

Extensive soft tissue mineralization of the stomach and intestines can suggest several causes. Renal failure resulting in uremia commonly leads to soft tissue mineralization. The mechanism is complex but involves tissue death and secondary mineralization. In guinea pigs, exposure to excessive vitamin D is a common mechanism if renal failure is not present.[29] Such exposure frequently occurs when feeding guinea pigs commercial rabbit pellets. Rabbit diets are formulated with more vitamin D than is safe for guinea pigs. Ingestion of some plants could also result in excessive vitamin D. These plants include many varieties such as *Cestrum diurnum, Trisetum flavescens*, and *Solanum malacoxylon*.[30]

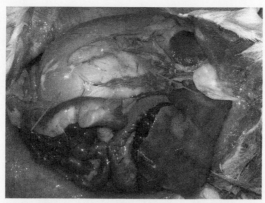

Fig. 5. The stomach is distended and torsed, resulting in displacement to the right side of the abdomen in this guinea pig. The *red arrows* indicate the stomach.

HAMSTERS
Gastrointestinal Tract

Bacteria

Hamster enteritis, also known as proliferative ileitis, transmissible ileal hyperplasia, and wet tail, can result in high morbidity as well as mortality. This is a most common and important disease. The cause is not completely determined, and multiple factors can affect the disease. It is frequently associated with a change in feed, housing, or husbandry practices in younger animals after weaning. It can present as acute, sub-acute, to chronic. The acute form results in death within 48 hours. The chronic form results in emaciated cachectic animals, with palpable ropey intestines. One common agent associated with this disease is a *Campylobacter*-like organism, *Lawsonia intracellularis*. The gross lesions are of thickening of the terminal ileum caused by hyperplasia of the crypt epithelium (**Fig. 6**).

Salmonella enteritides have all been caused by *Salmonella typhimurium*, which was serotyped to strains in concurrently infected children. The infections in hamsters resulted in unexpected death. On gross examination, there are fluid-filled and gas-filled small intestines and cecum. This infection is systemic, and the lungs also present with a patchy hemorrhagic grayish appearance with small white foci in the liver. These lesions are caused by bacteremia as well as thrombi, particularly to the lungs (**Fig. 7**).[1]

Protozoa

Giardiasis in hamsters ranges from subclinical to chronic wasting with diarrhea. The chronic form is associated with amyloidosis. The hamster protozoa are *Giardia muris* and their zoonotic significance is unknown.

Spironucleus (Hexamita) muris is common in some colonies of hamsters; it is found in small intestine and cecum and is considered nonpathogenic (**Fig. 8**).[1]

Metazoan

Hymenolepis nana (dwarf tapeworm) is the primary organism found in the small intestine of rats, mice, and hamsters. This common tapeworm has a direct and indirect life cycle. The clinical signs with heavy infestation include poor weight gains, abdominal distention, and diarrhea. The other cestode *Hymenolepis diminuta* infects hamsters with a moderate rate of incidence. Most adult rodents have developed immunity to these parasites (**Fig. 9**).

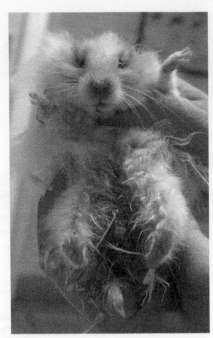

Fig. 6. The typical appearance of wet tail in a hamster. (*Courtesy of* Peter Fisher, DVM, Virginia Beach, VA.)

Hamsters are commonly infected with the mouse pinworm, *Syphacia obvelata*, although they have their own, *Syphacia mesocriceti*. The nematodes are generally found in the cecum and, to a lesser extent, colon. Syphacia has a direct life cycle, with eggs deposited around the anus. Mild enteritis may be associated with the infection.[1]

Miscellaneous
Antibiotic-associated colitis develops after treatment with antibiotics, particularly clindamycin. The normal bacterial flora are altered, and an overgrowth of *Clostridium*

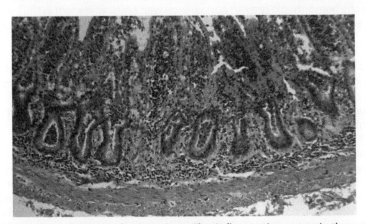

Fig. 7. *Salmonella* enteritis in the intestines. The inflammation extends throughout the mucosa (hematoxylin-eosin, original magnification ×40).

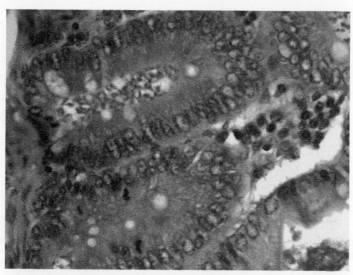

Fig. 8. Clusters of *Spironucleus* (*Hexamita*) *muris* (*red arrow*) within the lumen of the mucosal crypt. These bacteria are recognized in hamsters, mice, and rats (hematoxylin-eosin, original magnification ×400).

difficile is typical. There is a fatal colitis and, on gross examination, a distended food-filled cecum. The predominant bacterial flora of the hamster intestine are *Lactobacillus* and *Bacteroides*.

Intussusceptions have been reported in hamsters as a result of nutritional disturbances (**Fig. 10**). Intussusceptions also occur with existing or resolving enteritides. The clinical signs can include constipation.

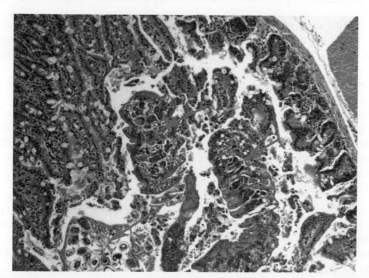

Fig. 9. *Hymenolepis* species (*red arrows*) within the intestinal lumen. These cestodes are common in hamsters, rats, and mice (hematoxylin-eosin, original magnification ×100).

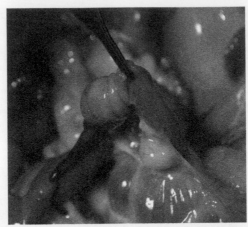

Fig. 10. Enteritis from many causes can result in intussusceptions. (*Courtesy of* Chris Griffin, DVM, Kannapolis, NC.)

Rectal prolapses are also common lesions of the digestive tract. Rectal prolapses have been induced by dietary changes or hypermotility associated with acute enteritis in hamsters. There is a dark red tubular protrusion from the anus. The prognosis is generally poor.[1]

Neoplasia
Intestinal carcinomas are occasionally described in hamsters. Some cases metastasized to the regional lymph nodes.[31]

MICE
Gastrointestinal Tract

Virus
Mouse hepatitis virus is one of the coronaviruses in mice. Many coronaviral strains, with varying virulence and organotropism, have been identified in mice. Those strains that have a primary tropism for enteric mucosa result in disease in mice less than 2 weeks of age or in immunocompromised mice. There is generally low mortality but high morbidity. The typical gross lesions are multifocal hepatic necrosis, icterus, ascites, and intestinal hemorrhage.

EDIM (epizootic diarrhea of infant mice) virus is caused by rotavirus and also has low mortality but high morbidity. The disease is present in mice infected at 12 or less days of age, and the lesions are of vacuolar degeneration of villus absorptive epithelium. Malabsorption, diarrhea, and runting are common clinical signs. The infection in older mice is subclinical.

Bacteria
The most common bacteria associated with gastroenteritis are *Citrobacter freundii*, *Clostridium piliforme* (Tyzzer disease), *Salmonella*, *Helicobacter*, and *Proteus*.

Transmissible murine colonic hyperplasia is associated with *Citrobacter freundii*. This infection results in low morbidity and mortality. Rectal prolapses are identified as well as runting. Thickening and rigidity of the distal colon are typical.[32]

Focal hepatic necrosis and enterocolitis are associated with Tyzzer disease in this species (*Clostridium piliforme*). Colitis with dissemination to liver (focal hepatitis) and occasionally heart (myocarditis) are the typical lesions. Special stains (silver, Giemsa, periodic acid-Schiff) can show intracytoplasmic bacteria.

Salmonella infections are a rare event and most infections are by *Salmonella enteritidis*. The bacteria invade Peyer patches of ileum and spread to the mesenteric lymph nodes, liver, and spleen.

Fungus

Gastric yeast is an incidental lesion identified in mice, hamsters, guinea pigs, gerbils, chinchillas, and rats. Morphologically, these yeast organisms appear consistent with *Candida albicans*. They have been identified in both glandular and squamous portions of the stomach (**Fig. 11**). They are typically associated with contaminated food or bedding.

Protozoan

Spironucleus (*Hexamita muris*) is frequently present in the alimentary tract of normal mice. This particular protozoon feeds on bacteria. Clinical disease, when it occurs, is in young animals at 3 to 6 weeks of age. There are predisposing factors. Clusters of the piriform protozoa accumulate along the mucosa of the intestines and can be seen associated with a neutrophilic enteritis.

Giardia muris is a flagellate that normally resides in the duodenum lumen. Mice are the natural hosts.

Coccidiosis is an uncommon protozoal disease in young mice. When clinical signs are noted, there is bloody diarrhea and runting of juvenile animals. Several *Eimeria* species have been described in murine intestinal infections, although *Eimeria falciformis* is most common. Lesions have been more commonly recognized in the large intestine and are associated with diffuse subacute colitis (**Fig. 12**).

Cryptosporidium muris and *Cryptosporidium parvum* are infections recognized in young poor-doing mice, generally suffering multiple diseases. In mice, *Cryptosporidium parvum* colonizes the upper small intestine and *Cryptosporidium muris* is within the stomach. Both are mildly pathogenic and lead to malnutrition (**Fig. 13**).

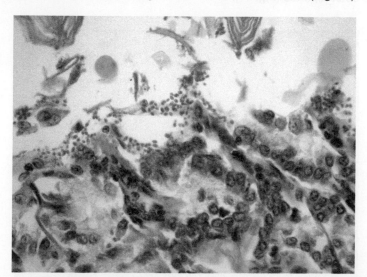

Fig. 11. Clusters of oval yeast are massed along the border of the mucosa of the glandular stomach. This condition has been reported in mice, hamsters, guinea pigs, gerbils, chinchillas, and rats (hematoxylin-eosin, original magnification ×400).

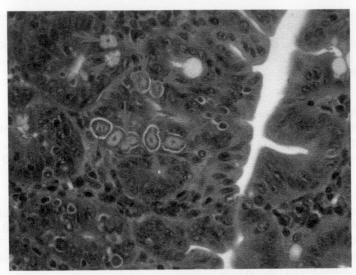

Fig. 12. *Coccidia* (*red arrows*) in various stages of development within the enterocytes (hematoxylin-eosin, original magnification ×400).

Metazoan

Syphacia obvelata and *Aspicularis tetraptera* (pinworms) nematodes are generally found in the cecum and, to a lesser extent, in the colon. *Syphacia* has a direct life cycle, with eggs (banana shaped) deposited around the anus. A mild enteritis may be associated with the infection, and many cases also have a perineal dermatitis. *Aspicularis* does not deposit eggs (symmetrically shaped) around the anus. Resistance to infection develops with age. Treatment is generally unrewarding. Rectal prolapse has been reported (**Fig. 14**).

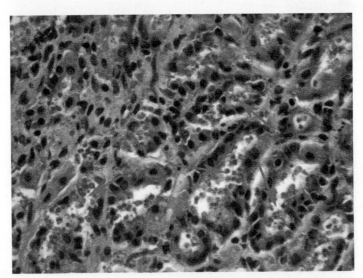

Fig. 13. Cryptosporidia are proliferating along the cytoplasmic borders of the lining mucosal epithelium (*red arrows*) (hematoxylin-eosin, original magnification ×40).

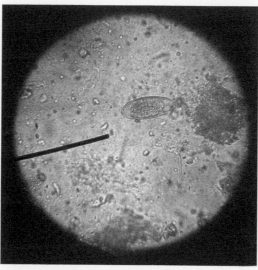

Fig. 14. The egg of *Syphacia* (pinworm) in a fecal float from a mouse. (*Courtesy of* Peter Fisher, DVM, Virginia Beach, VA.)

Heavy infestation with *Hymenolepis nana*, *Hymenolepis diminuta*, and *Hymenolepis microstoma* is associated with poor weight gains, abdominal distention, and diarrhea. *Hymenolepis nana* (dwarf tapeworm) is the primary organism found in the small intestine of rats, mice, and hamster. *Hymenolepis nana* is considered zoonotic. Most adult rodents develop an immunity to these parasites.

Neoplasia
Odontomas are rarely described in mice. Odontomas include ameloblastic fibro-odontoma[33] and a bilateral complex odontoma.[34]

Adenocarcinoma has been reported in the colon of mice.[35]

RABBIT
Oral Disease

Edematous to erythematous macules or papules around the mouth and on the lips are the typical lesions of acute rabbit syphilis. The cause is *Treponema cuniculi*, a helical rod-shaped bacterium that has the ability to penetrate intact mucous membranes.[36,37] The lesions also develop on the vulva and prepuce, anus, nose, scrotum, eyelids, and base of the ears. More chronic lesions appear as crusty ulcerative sores (**Fig. 15**). On histologic examination, there are epidermal acanthosis, erosions and ulcerations, microabscesses or vesicle formation, and a dermal infiltrate of numerous plasma cells and macrophages. Special stains may be necessary to identify the *Treponema* organism. This organism is spread primarily horizontally during breeding of adults. It may also be spread vertically from dam to offspring during vaginal delivery or suckling.

An oral papillomatosis virus has been identified in young rabbits.[38,39] Lesions involve the nonkeratinized mucous epithelial surfaces. These lesions are present primarily on the ventral aspect of the tongue, especially in areas abraded by maloccluded teeth (**Fig. 16**). They are typically solitary papillary growths, which regress. On histologic examination, there may be small basophilic intranuclear inclusions within the stratum spinosum, consistent with rabbit oral papillomavirus.

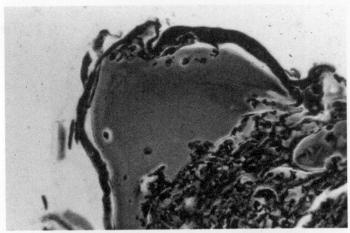

Fig. 15. A silver stain highlights the thin, spiral bacteria of *Treponema cuniculi* (Grocott methenamine silver, original magnification ×400).

Gastrointestinal Tract

Bacteria

Small intestinal proliferative enteritis in the domestic rabbit presents with soft, watery diarrhea, which often contains mucus and blood.[40,41] The rabbits, primarily weanlings, have distention and mucosal thickening of the small intestine, with enlarged mesenteric lymph nodes. The histologic appearance includes an infiltrate of macrophages

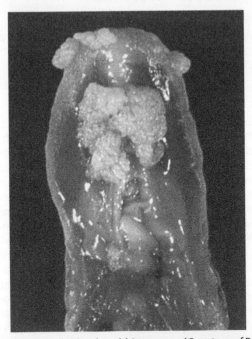

Fig. 16. Papilloma on the ventral side of a rabbit tongue. (*Courtesy of* Robert Schmidt, DVM, Anthem, AZ.)

and lymphocytes and a mucosa thickened with elongated tortuous and sometimes branched crypts. One report identified an uncharacterized bacterium in apical cytoplasm. Warthin-Starry stains in another report identified numerous rod-shaped to spiral bacteria in the apical cytoplasm. This bacterium morphologically is consistent with *Lawsonia intracellularis*, the cause of proliferative enteropathy in other species.

Protozoa

Intestinal coccidiosis, which uncommonly results in disease, can be diagnosed with a fecal parasitic examination. Occasionally, an ulcerative enterocolitis is described. Hepatic and biliary *Coccidia*, which are uncommon in other animal species, are common in domestic and wild rabbits. *Eimeria stiedae* is the *Coccidia* of rabbits. There may be clinical signs with heavy infestations, although young rabbits may experience some mortality. On gross examination, the liver is generally enlarged, with multiple raised firm, yellow-white to gray lesions on the surface. The cut surface may have enlarged bile ducts, which are thickened, fibrotic, and dilated, and occasionally filled with green bile and debris. The liver has a chronic proliferative cholangitis with biliary ectasia. A lymphoplasmacytic periportal infiltrate may be recognized. This condition may resolve to portal fibrosis and bile duct hyperplasia.

Miscellaneous

Intestinal smooth muscle hypertrophy presents as a uniform hypertrophy of the smooth muscle tunics in the intestinal section, with mild mucosal hypertrophy. No cause for this disease has been determined, although similar intestinal stenotic lesions have been described in young dogs, cats, and horses.

Mucosal rectoanal papilloma is an uncommonly reported lesion in rabbits. It has been described primarily in older male rabbits and shown to be nonviral in origin. These papillomas are usually well-differentiated growths, and the few cases reported have been benign (**Fig. 17**). Complete surgical removal is recommended, because these lesions are reported to undergo neoplastic transformation in other mammalian species.

Neoplasia

Of the neoplastic diseases, lymphoma is most frequently identified within the liver. Other reported locations include the gastric fundus, the spleen, mesenteric lymph

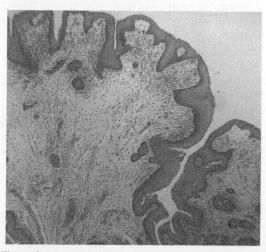

Fig. 17. Rectal papilloma from a rabbit (hematoxylin-eosin, original magnification ×400).

nodes, bone marrow, pulmonary interstitium, and adrenal glands. In some reports, this disease is considered to be the second most commonly occurring neoplastic condition.[42] Lymphomas in rabbits are usually associated with an aleukemic hematologic profile. The neoplasm is most commonly seen in juvenile and young adult rabbits. Histologic appearance is of infiltration and effacement of the normal architecture by neoplastic lymphocytes.

RAT
Oral Disease

The long rat incisors can be broken or trimmed too short by caretakers, resulting in dental disease and inflammation/infection of the surrounding soft tissues. If foreign material from feedstuffs or caging materials becomes impacted in the pulp cavity and the periodontal space, this may lead to endodontitis or periodontitis.

Gastrointestinal Tract

Bacteria
Tyzzer disease, caused by *Clostridium piliforme* (formerly known as *Bacillus piliformis*) results in a unique dilation of the terminal small intestine of rats. This particular bacterial infection has a wide host range, which includes rats, hamsters, and guinea pigs. There is generally low morbidity but high mortality. Other lesions include focal areas of hepatic necrosis.

Metazoan
Rats serve as intermediate hosts for the cat tapeworm *Taenia taeniaeformis*. Rats, mice, and hamsters ingest the eggs, which hatch and migrate through the bowel and encyst in the liver. The cysticercoid cyst (*Cysticercus fasciolaris*) embeds in the liver and may develop large cysts.

Miscellaneous
Gastric ulceration and erosions can be identified in the glandular or nonglandular region. There is generally no specific cause, although these conditions are not uncommonly associated with a stress response or trauma from gavage feeding.

Neoplasia
Several variations of odontoma have been described in rats. These tumors consist of cementum, dentin, enamel, and pulp tissue, which may be arranged in the form of teeth. Odontomas are further divided according to morphologic features and degree of organization. A complex odontoma and an ameloblastic odontoma have both been recognized.[43,44]

One gastric carcinoid tumor developed in the glandular stomach of an older rat. It appeared as a focal raised mass.[45]

Colonic adenocarcinoma has been described many times in the literature. These lesions appear as constrictions typically just below the ileocecal junction (proximal colon). The tumor mass fills the lumen of the colon. Mucosal ulceration and metastases to adjacent lymph nodes or local implantation on serosal surfaces are commonly associated lesions.[46–48] There has been 1 report of a gelatinous carcinoma of the cecum.[46]

SUGAR GLIDER
Gastrointestinal Tract

Bacteria
From the author's review, acute to subacute enteritis and colitis are common lesions. These lesions are usually associated with inflammatory lesions in the liver, heart,

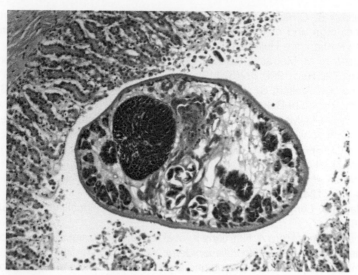

Fig. 18. A trematode within the lumen of the stomach (hematoxylin-eosin, original magnification ×100).

kidney, and brain. Specific microbes are seldom recognized, and many cases are suspected to be caused by endotoxemias. A common history is of unexpected death, occasionally with terminal neurologic clinical signs.

Clostridium piliforme has been reported. Giardiasis and cryptosporidia are also described as a cause of diarrhea.[49] All these causes have been described previously.

Metazoan
Intestinal metazoans are rarely reported in sugar gliders. The author has identified gastrointestinal trematodiasis. The trematodes were identified as from the genus *Plagiorchis* and were associated with enteritis (**Fig. 18**).

Miscellaneous
Gastric dilatation and volvulus was diagnosed in 2 adult sugar gliders presenting for acute illness featuring abdominal distention. Confirmation was made at necropsy. Histopathology of multiple tissues showed several underlying disease conditions, but gave no specific direct cause.[50]

Neoplasia
There is scant literature about neoplasia in sugar gliders. One pericloacal transitional cell carcinoma resulted in severe cloacal narrowing and intestinal distention. The tumor arose from the urothelium of the urethra and urinary bladder and encompassed the colon and cloaca.[51]

REFERENCES

1. Reavill DR. The pathology of common diseases in small exotic mammals. AVCP 2004. Proceedings on CD at Charles Louis Davis, DVM Foundation. Available at: http://www.afip.org/CLDavis/index.html. Accessed December 2008.
2. Legendre LF. Malocclusions in guinea pigs, chinchillas and rabbits. Can Vet J 2002;43(5):385–90.

3. Boehmer E, Crossley D. Objective interpretation of dental disease in rabbits, guinea pigs and chinchillas. Use of anatomical reference lines. Tierarztl Prax Ausg K Klientiere Heimtiere 2009;37(4):250–60.
4. Bartoszcze M, Matras J, Palec S, et al. *Klebsiella pneumoniae* infection in chinchillas. Vet Rec 1990;127(5):119.
5. Wuthe HH, Aleksia S. *Yersinia enterocolitica* serovar 1,2a,3 biovar 3 in chinchillas. Zentralbl Bakteriol 1992;277(3):403–5.
6. Wilkerson MJ, Melendy A, Stauber E. An outbreak of listeriosis in a breeding colony of chinchillas. J Vet Diagn Invest 1997;9:320–3.
7. Wood JS, Bennett IV, Yardley JH. Staphylococcal enterocolitis in chinchillas. Bull Johns Hopkins Hosp 1956;98(6):454–63.
8. Larrivee GP, Elvehjem CA. Disease problems in chinchillas. J Am Vet Med Assoc 1954;124(927):447–55.
9. Finley GG, Long JR. An epizootic of listeriosis in chinchillas. Can Vet J 1977; 18(6):164–7.
10. Kimpe A, Decostere A, Hermans K, et al. Isolation of *Listeria ivanovii* from a septicaemic chinchilla (*Chinchilla lanigera*). Vet Rec 2004;154(25):791–2.
11. Yamini B, Raju NR. Gastroenteritis associated with a *Cryptosporidium* sp in a chinchilla. J Am Vet Med Assoc 1986;189(9):1158–9.
12. Levecke B, Meulemans L, Dalemans T, et al. Mixed *Giardia duodenalis* assemblage A, B, C and E infections in pet chinchillas (*Chinchilla lanigera*) in Flanders (Belgium). Vet Parasitol 2011;177(1–2):166–70.
13. Shelton GC. Giardiasis in the chinchilla. I. Observations on morphology, location in the intestinal tract, and host specificity. Am J Vet Res 1954;15(54):71–4.
14. Veronesi F, Fioretti DP, Morganti G, et al. Occurrence of *Giardia duodenalis* infection in chinchillas (*Chinchilla lanigera*) from Italian breeding facilities. Res Vet Sci 2012;93(2):807–10.
15. Olsen OW. Natural infection of chinchillas with the mouse tapeworm, *Hymenolepis nana* var. fraternal. Vet Med 1950;45(11):440–2.
16. Bartoszce M, Nowakowska M, Roszkowski J, et al. Chinchilla deaths due to *Clostridium perfringens* A enterotoxin. Vet Rec 1990;126(14):341–2.
17. Moore RW, Greenlee HH. Enterotoxaemia in chinchillas. Lab Anim 1975;9(2): 153–4.
18. Jenkins JR. Diseases of geriatric guinea pigs and chinchillas. Veterinary Clin North Am Exot Anim Pract 2010;13(1):85–93.
19. Smith JL, Campbell-Ward M, Else RW, et al. Undifferentiated carcinoma of the salivary gland in a chinchilla (*Chinchilla lanigera*). J Vet Diagn Invest 2010; 22(1):152–5.
20. Lucena RB, Rissi DR, Queiroz DM, et al. Infiltrative gastric adenocarcinoma in a chinchilla (*Chinchilla lanigera*). J Vet Diagn Invest 2012;24(4):797–800.
21. Nambiar PR, Kirchain S, Fox JG. Gastritis-associated adenocarcinoma and intestinal metaplasia in a Syrian hamster naturally infected with *Helicobacter* species. Vet Pathol 2005;42:386–93.
22. Watanabe T, Tada M, Nagai H, et al. *Helicobacter pylori* induces gastric cancer in Mongolian gerbils. Gastroenterology 1998;115(3):642–8.
23. Vincent GP, Pare WP. Activity-stress ulcer in the rat, hamster, gerbil and guinea pig. Physiol Behav 1976;16(5):557–60.
24. Rowe SE, Simmons JL, Ringler DH, et al. Spontaneous neoplasms in aging Gerbillinae. A summary of forty-four neoplasms. Vet Pathol 1974;11(1):38–51.
25. Meckley PE, Zwicker GM. Naturally-occurring neoplasms in the Mongolian gerbil, *Meriones unguiculatus*. Lab Anim 1979;13(3):203–6.

26. Vincent AL, Ash LR. Further observations on spontaneous neoplasms in the Mongolian gerbil, *Meriones unguiculatus*. Lab Anim Sci 1978;28(3): 297–300.

27. Guzman-Silva MA. Systemic mast cell disease in the Mongolian gerbil, *Meriones unguiculatus*: case report. Lab Anim 1997;31(4):373–8.

28. Olfert ED, Ward GE, Stevenson D. *Salmonella typhimurium* infection in guinea pigs: observations on monitoring and control. Lab Anim Sci 1976;26(1): 78–80.

29. Kruckenberg SM, Cook JE, Feldman BF. Clinical toxicities of pet and caged rodents and rabbits. Vet Clin North Am 1975;5(4):675–84.

30. Sparschu GL, Christie RJ. Metastatic calcification in a guinea pig colony: a pathological survey. Lab Anim Care 1968;18(5):520–6.

31. Jelinek F. Adenocarcinomas of the small intestine in golden hamsters. Z Versuchstierkd 1986;28(3):153–5.

32. Barthold SW, Coleman GL, Jacoby RO, et al. Transmissible murine colonic hyperplasia. Vet Pathol 1978;27:223–36.

33. Nyska A, Waner T, Tal H, et al. Spontaneous ameloblastic fibro-odontoma in a female mouse. J Oral Pathol Med 1991;20(5):250–2.

34. Dayan D, Waner T, Harmelin A, et al. Bilateral complex odontoma in a Swiss (CD-1) male mouse. Lab Anim 1994;28(1):90–2.

35. Madarame H, Sakurai H. Spontaneous adenocarcinoma of the colon in a DDD mouse. Lab Anim Sci 1993;43(1):108–10.

36. Cunliffe-Beamer TL, Fox RR. Venereal spirochetosis of rabbits: description and diagnosis, epizootiology, eradication. (3 articles). Lab Anim Sci 1981;31(4): 366–71, 372–8, 379–81.

37. DiGiacomo RF. *Treponema paraluis-cuniculi* infection in a commercial rabbitry: epidemiology and serodiagnosis. Lab Anim Sci 1983;33(6):562–6.

38. Sundberg JP, Junge RE, el Shazly MO. Oral papillomatosis in New Zealand white rabbits. Am J Vet Res 1985;46(3):664–8.

39. Weisbroth SH, Scher S. Spontaneous oral papilloma in rabbits. J Am Vet Med Assoc 1970;157:1940–4.

40. Umemura T, Tsuchitani M, Totsuka M, et al. Histiocytic enteritis of rabbits. Vet Pathol 1981;18:326–9.

41. Hotchkiss CE, Shames B, Perkins SE, et al. Proliferative enteropathy of rabbits: the intracellular *Campylobacter*-like organism is closely related to *Lawsonia intracellularis*. Lab Anim Sci 1996;46(6):623–7.

42. Cloyd GG, Johnson GR. Lymphosarcoma with lymphoblastic leukemia in a New Zealand white rabbit. Lab Anim Sci 1978;28(1):66–9.

43. Jang DD, Kim CK, Ahn B, et al. Spontaneous complex odontoma in a Sprague-Dawley rat. J Vet Med Sci 2002;64(3):289–91.

44. Barbolt TA, Bhandari JC. Ameloblastic odontoma in a rat. Lab Anim Sci 1983; 33(6):583–4.

45. Majka JA, Sher S. Spontaneous gastric carcinoid tumor in an aged Sprague-Dawley rat. Vet Pathol 1989;26(1):88–90.

46. Burn JI, Sellwood RA, Bishop M. Spontaneous carcinoma of the colon of the rat. J Pathol Bacteriol 1966;91(1):253–4.

47. Grasso P, Creasey M. Carcinoma of the colon in a rat. Eur J Cancer 1969;5(4): 415–9.

48. Miwa M, Takenaka S, Ito K, et al. Spontaneous colon tumors in rats. J Natl Cancer Inst 1976;56(3):615–21.

49. Brust DM. Sugar gliders. Exotic DVM 2009;11(3):32–41.

50. Lennox AM, Reavill DR. Gastric dilatation and gastric dilatation with volvulus in two sugar gliders (*Petaurus breviceps*). Proceedings of Association of Exotic Mammal Veterinarians. Indianapolis (IN); 2013. p. 21–22.

51. Marrow JC, Carpenter JW, Lloyd A, et al. A Transitional cell carcinoma with squamous differentiation in a pericloacal mass in a sugar glider (*Petaurus breviceps*). J Exotic Pet Med 2010;19(1):92–5.

Gastrointestinal Anatomy and Physiology of Select Exotic Companion Mammals

Micah Kohles, DVM, MPA[a,b,*]

KEYWORDS

- Rabbits • Guinea pigs • Chinchillas • Small herbivores • Fiber • Hindgut
- Gastrointestinal • Cecotroph • Colonic separation mechanism

KEY POINTS

- The anatomy and gastrointestinal physiology of rabbits, guinea pigs, and chinchillas are different from those of other exotic companion mammals.
- Rabbits, guinea pigs, and chinchillas are all concentrate selectors, hindgut fermenters, and coprophagic.
- They are designed to intake large quantities of high-fibrous, low-energy-density foods.
- They use unique colonic separation mechanisms and have open-rooted, constantly growing dentition.
- Gastrointestinal disease, often secondary to diet or environmental factors, is common in these species.

INTRODUCTION

The anatomy and gastrointestinal physiology of rabbits, guinea pigs, and chinchillas are different from those of other exotic companion mammals. These species are strict herbivores, classified as hindgut (cecum and colon) fermenters and concentrate selectors, and are designed to ingest large amounts of high-fibrous food. As prey species, maintaining a small body size is advantageous. Their unique gastrointestinal system, with its rapid transit time and ability to differentiate particulates of fiber, allows them to remain small and active, while surviving on high-fiber, low-energy-density plant materials. Although all 3 species have similar gastrointestinal function and nutritional needs, each has some unique species traits. Gastrointestinal disease in these species is a very common presenting issue in clinical practice. It is often associated with dysbiosis and can present as both primary and secondary disease.

Disclosure: This article originally appeared in similar form in the proceedings of the 2013 Association of Exotic Mammal Veterinarians Conference in Indianapolis, Indiana, USA.
[a] Oxbow Animal Health, 29012 Mill Road Murdock, Nebraska, NE 68407, USA; [b] School of Veterinary Medicine and Biomedical Sciences, University of Nebraska-Lincoln Lincoln, Nebraska, NE 68583, USA
* Oxbow Animal Health, 29012 Mill Road Murdock, Nebraska, NE 68407.
E-mail address: mkohles@oxbowanimalhealth.com

RABBIT

Domestic rabbits (*Oryctolagus cuniculus*) are herbivores and concentrate selectors, and are classified as hindgut (cecum and colon) fermenters. They are mostly crepuscular and nocturnal feeders. They are anatomically and physiologically adapted to handle significant amounts of low-energy-density fibrous food and to effectively use the nutrients found in a high-fiber diet (**Fig. 1**). However, because of their small body size they are unable to store large amounts of food material and therefore use

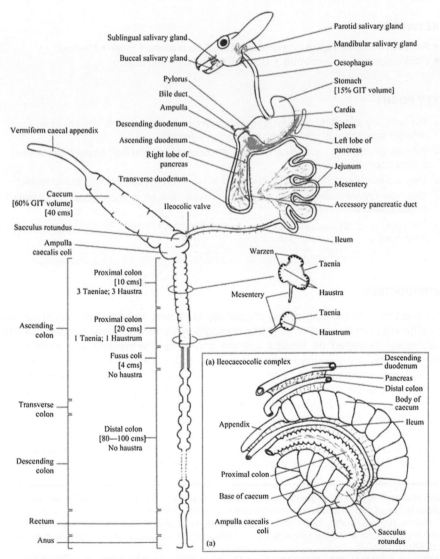

Fig. 1. Schematic diagram of the anatomy of the alimentary tract of the rabbit. cms, Centimeters; GIT, Gastrointestinal Tract; HCO3, Bicarbonate; H⁺CL, Hydrochloric Acid; VFA, Volatile Fatty Acids. (*From* Harcourt-Brown F. Biologic characteristics of the domestic rabbit (*Oryctolagus cuniculi*). In: Harcourt-Brown F, editor. Textbook of Rabbit Medicine. Burlington (VT): Butterworth-Heinemann; 2002. p. 1–18; with permission.)

a unique process to rapidly eliminate fiber for the gastrointestinal system. Their gastrointestinal system allows for the intake of large amounts of low-energy-density, high-fiber food that is separated based on particle size. The easily fermentable component of the diet is retained, whereas the slowly fermentable components of the diet (preeminently cellulose-based plant fiber) are rapidly eliminated. This separation process allows for the production of 2 types of stool: a dry, hard, high-fiber fecal pellet and an enlarged, soft fecal pellet that is covered in mucous and referred to as a cecotrope (eg, cecal, night stool). Rabbits, like all herbivores, have a symbiotic relationship with a diversity of gut flora (primarily *Bacteroides*), because they lack mammalian enzymes to break down the cellulose components of their plant-based diets. Some of the most common health issues with domestic rabbits, both in companion and commercial animals, are related to the gastrointestinal system. The symbiotic relationship rabbits have with the microflora in the cecum allows them to effectively ferment plant structural carbohydrates, which provide their main energy source.

Ingestion of Food

Rabbits have a large cornea and laterally placed eyes, which give them a panoramic field of view when grazing and foraging. Food is selected based on smell and tactile perception of the lips, because their visual field does not include the area just under their nose.[1] As concentrate selectors, rabbits will choose the most tender, succulent plant parts, which are nutrient-dense and lowest in fiber to meet their nutritional needs owing to a high metabolic rate. Rabbits have open-rooted (constantly growing) incisor and cheek teeth.

Rabbits' incisors are designed to apprehend and cut through vegetation. The large upper incisors have 2 smaller incisors behind them (peg teeth). The occlusion of the upper and lower incisors allows the teeth to be constantly sharpened. The premolar and molar teeth, also known as *cheek teeth*, are designed to process hard fibrous foods. The fibrous food is ground between the cheek teeth with jaw movements up to 120 per minute.[1] This repetitive, rapid chewing movement maintains proper dental health. It should be noted that when rabbits ingest cecotrophs, normal mastication does not occur and the cecotrophs are swallowed intact.[2] When a rabbit is fed an unsuitable diet, such as low-fiber muesli mixes and minimal or no hay, improper dental wear can quickly occur, leading to dental disease. A suitable diet of high-fiber hay and high-fiber uniform pellets will help control the growth of the teeth and prevent overgrowth and malocclusion. As concentrate selectors, rabbits, like deer, have a predisposition to select the lower-fiber, more tender portions of their diets, which, if they are fed cereal-based or mixed pellets, can lead to selective feeding and malnutrition.

If low-fiber mixed cereal or seed-based foods are eaten, the rapid chewing activity is no longer required, which can result in dental disease, such as malocclusion and clinical and/or reserve crown elongation, and a multitude of potential gastrointestinal issues. As the teeth elongate, secondary to inadequate wear, the jaws are forced apart and the radiographic appearance of the diastema increases. Over time, the upper and lower jaws begin to no longer occlude properly and mandibular movement is reduced. The condition deteriorates as the teeth become mobile and maloccluded, resulting in the development of spurs that may lacerate and ulcerate the tongue and buccal cavity. These punctures or lacerations are painful to the rabbit and may result in secondary infection from bacterial invasion of the tongue or other soft tissues of the mouth.

Stomach

The stomach of the rabbit is J-shaped and large compared with most monogastrics, constitutes roughly 15% of the gastrointestinal tract, has a well-developed cardiac sphincter that prevents vomiting, and a muscular pyloric area.[1,3] The rabbit stomach is divided into 4 parts (the cardia, fundus, body, and pylorus) and contains numerous folds, called *rugae*. The cardia is large, thin-walled, nonglandular, and lined with stratified squamous epithelium.[4] The pH of the stomach is low and ranges from 1 to 6. The pH is affected by a variety of factors, including the location where pH is measured, the presence or absence of soft feces, the duration of time from feed intake, and the age of the rabbit.[5] The pH of weanling rabbits is higher (5.0–6.5), which permits the passage of bacteria through the stomach to the hindgut to colonize the cecum.[1]

The inner mucosa of the stomach is lined with gastric glands that secrete hydrochloric acid and the enzyme pepsinogen to begin the process of protein digestion.[6] The stomach transit time is between 3 and 6 hours.[5] The stomach acts as a holding chamber, should always contain ingesta, and has been shown after a 24-hour fast to still be 50% full, usually with a mass of food material and hair surrounded by fluid.[7] Trichobezoars (hairballs) were originally believed to be caused by fur ingestion but are now believed to be associated with decreased gastric movement, potentially because of reduced intestinal motility and/or physical inactivity of the rabbit.[1] Captive rabbits kept in cages face the potential challenges of inadequate exercise and obesity, which can be negative factors related to gastrointestinal health.

Small Intestinal Tract

The rabbit small intestine, made up of the duodenum, jejunum (longest), and ileum, is short compared with that of other species, at approximately 3 m in length, and constitutes approximately 12% of the total gastrointestinal tract.[4] Transit time through the jejunum and ileum is 10 to 20 and 30 to 60 minutes, respectively.[5] The duodenum is the largest of 3 segments but shortest in length (3–5 inches in rabbits).[6] The bile duct and pancreatic duct enter the duodenum separately, with the bile duct entering proximal to the pancreatic duct.[4] The jejunum is less vascularized and its walls are thinner than those of the duodenum.[4] The distal end of the ileum is thickened and referred to as the sacculus rotundus, which marks the intersection of the ileum, colon and cecum. This location signals the beginning of the large intestine and links to the ampulla coli, which form an intersection of the distal ileum, cecum, and proximal colon. The sacculus rotundus (**Fig. 2**) is unique to the rabbit and has abundant

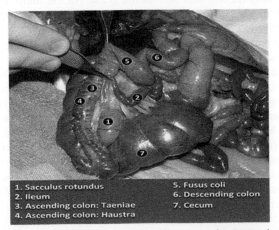

1. Sacculus rotundus
2. Ileum
3. Ascending colon: Taeniae
4. Ascending colon: Haustra
5. Fusus coli
6. Descending colon
7. Cecum

Fig. 2. Rabbit hind gut and distal small intestine. (*Courtesy of* K. Rosenthal, DVM, West Bay, Cayman Islands.)

aggregations of lymphoid tissue and macrophages in the lamina propria and submucosa.[1] It is also within the ileum that Peyer patches first appear. Located at the junction of the ileum and the large intestine is the ileocecal valve, which regulates the movement of material from the small intestine into the large intestine and prevents the retrograde movement of intestinal contents.

The small intestine is the site where the greater part of digestion and absorption occurs during passive and active transportation throughout the mucosa.[5] The stomach and small intestine in rabbits digest and absorb nutrients similarly to those in monogastric animals, with hydrochloric acid and pepsin as initiators of digestion, whereas pancreatic enzyme production, such as amylase, is minimal, with most coming from saliva or bacterial production within the cecotroph.[1] Most digestion of carbohydrates and simple proteins occurs in the duodenum and jejunum, and the products are absorbed across the jejunal brush border.[8] Motilin, a polypeptide hormone secreted by enterochromaffin cells of the duodenum and jejunum, stimulates gastrointestinal smooth muscle. Motilin activity decreases in the distal small intestine and is absent in the cecum, but reappears in the colon and rectum.[8] Motilin production is stimulated by fat and inhibited by carbohydrate ingestion.[1] The transit time of the rabbit small intestine is rapid compared with that of other herbivorous species, and fiber is quickly moved to the cecum and large intestine.

A key function of this component of a rabbit's gastrointestinal system is the digestion of cecotrophs. Cecotrophs are soft, dark colored contents of the cecum that are rich in bacteria, amino acids, vitamins, and minerals.[1] They are expelled rapidly from the cecum (1.5–2.5 times faster than hard feces) through the colon, without undergoing any separation, and therefore maintain a higher moisture content than typically feces. They are coated in a protective mucous, which protects them from the acidity of the stomach, to allow for continued bacterial fermentation before absorption in the small intestine. Microbial protein is an important source of amino acids for rabbits, and lysozyme, an enzyme added in the colon, allows for the degradation of microbial protein. Increased levels of fiber intake increase cecotroph production, whereas high protein intake levels reduce it.[1]

Hindgut Cecum/Colon

The rabbit cecum is very large and has a capacity roughly 10 times that of the stomach, constituting around 40% of the total gastrointestinal tract.[3] It is a thin-walled organ that folds on itself multiple times and has an internal surface composed of a long spiral fold (sometimes referred to as *spiral valve*) that is continued into the beginning of the colon, an area known as the *ampulla coli*. The distal tip of the cecum is known as the vermiform appendix. This tube-like area is narrow and thickened and contains significant amounts of lymphoid aggregates, which secrete bicarbonate ions into the cecum. These bicarbonate ions act as a buffering agent for the volatile fatty acids formed during cecal fermentation.[2] Rabbits fed diets low in fiber and high in fermentable carbohydrates develop an enlarged appendix.[8] It has been hypothesized that this provides evidence that increased appendix secretory function is needed to counteract the products of increased carbohydrate fermentation.[8]

The colon of the rabbit is divided into 3 sections: the ascending, transverse, and descending colon. The fusus coli (located anatomically at the transverse colon) forms a natural division between the morphologically and functionally distinct ascending and descending sections of the rabbit colon. Many physiology textbooks have abandoned the 3-section description of the rabbit colon, and simplify using the terms *proximal* and *distal colon*.[1,9] The colon is a very functional component of the hindgut and is characterized by sacculations (haustra) and bands (taeniae). The ascending colon has 4 sections that contain small luminal protrusions, approximately 0.5 mm in diameter, which are commonly referred to as *warzens*. These wart-like protrusions are believed to be unique to rabbits. They potentially represent an increase in the surface area of the colon that would favor absorption and also may assist in mechanical separation of gut contents.[1] The number of taeniae and haustra gradually taper throughout the proximal colon to the point of the fusus coli, where they are absent. The fusus coli has a mucosa that is 4 to 5 times thicker than the descending colon and contains ganglion aggregates.[1] The fusus coli is commonly referred to as the "pacemaker" of the hind gut and controls the retrograde and normograde peristaltic activities that occur during the formation of soft and hard feces. The autonomic nervous system and adrenal glands may participate in the regulation of the fusus, which may explain why rabbits are prone to stress-related gastrointestinal disease (as opposed to this being due to immunosuppression).[1] The descending colon mucosa is smooth and, although it contains numerous goblet cells, does not contain obvious specialization and usually contains hard fecal pellets.[1] Gut-associated lymphoid tissue and specialized cells (goblet or Paneth cells, responsible for mucous and antimicrobial peptide secretion, respectively) regulate the interaction of the gut mucosa with the microbiota and develop mechanisms of tolerance and protection against pathogens.[5]

Rabbit Hindgut Physiology

The rhythmic contractions of the cecum constantly mix the ingesta as it undergoes fermentation by the mixed bacterial population, predominantly *Bacteroides* spp. The effects of bacterial fermentation include the production of volatile fatty acids (VFAs), including acetic, formic, propionic, and butyric acids, which are a major energy source in rabbits. A portion of these VFAs are contained in cecotrophs and used on reingestion, whereas another portion is absorbed directly across the cecal mucosa. Rabbits differ from other animals in that the level of butyric acid normally exceeds that of propionic acids, with proportions of VFA in the cecum contents being 60% to 70% acetic, 15% to 20% butyric, and 10% to 15% propionic acid.[5]

An almost continuous flux of material occurs between the cecum and the proximal colon ("wash back"). The mixture of fluid and nutrients is moved through vigorous peristalsis in normograde and retrograde directions (**Fig. 3**). These contractions result in large indigestible fibrous particles accumulating in the center of the colon, where they are rapidly transported in a normograde direction along the colon to the rectum for defecation. Water, electrolytes, and VFAs are removed from the contents as they move normograde towards excretion. Conversely, smaller more fermentable fibrous particles and fluids accumulate at the periphery of the colon where, through retrograde peristaltic contractions of the haustra, they are returned to the cecum for further fermentation.

Periodically, a dramatic change occurs in the peristaltic activity of the cecum and colon as the retrograde movement of smaller fiber particles ceases and a large quantity of the cecal content is expelled into the colon. These contents are excreted, usually once to twice daily, as soft, mucous-covered cecotrophs, beginning approximately 4 hours after food ingestion. This process is controlled by the fusus coli. The ability of the colon to rapidly eliminate large indigestible fiber particles and retain smaller more digestible fiber for further fermentation makes the rabbit an extremely efficient herbivore, capable of surviving on very low-quality forage.

The cecotroph fermentation process depends heavily on an appropriate diet and the action of resident bacteria (especially *Bacteroides* spp) and protozoa, which are vital to the gastrointestinal health of the rabbit. Dysbiosis is a common sequela of gastrointestinal disease and, owing to the importance of microbial function in hindgut

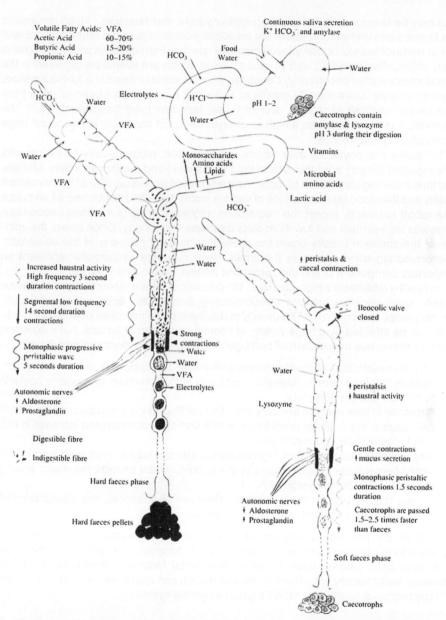

Volatile Fatty Acids: VFA
Acetic Acid   60–70%
Butyric Acid   15–20%
Propionic Acid   10–15%

HCO₃

Continuous saliva secretion
K⁺ HCO₃⁻ and amylase

Food
Water

Water

HCO₃
Water

Electrolytes

H⁺Cl⁻

pH 1–2

Water

VFA

Caecotrophs contain
amylase & lysozyme
pH 3 during their digestion

Water

Monosaccharides
Amino acids
Lipids

VFA

HCO₃⁻

VFA

Vitamins

Microbial
amino acids

Lactic acid

Water

Increased haustral activity
High frequency 3 second
duration contractions

Segmental low frequency
14 second duration
contractions

Monophasic progressive
peristaltic wave
5 seconds duration

Autonomic nerves
↑ Aldosterone
↑ Prostaglandin

Digestible fibre

Indigestible fibre

Hard faeces phase

Hard faeces pellets

Strong
contractions
Water

Water

VFA

Electrolytes

Water

↑ peristalsis &
caecal contraction

Ileocolic valve
closed

Water

Lysozyme

↑ peristalsis
↓ haustral activity

Autonomic nerves
↑ Aldosterone
↑ Prostaglandin

Gentle contractions
↑ mucus secretion

Monophasic peristaltic
contractions 1.5 seconds
duration

Caecotrophs are passed
1.5–2.5 times faster
than faeces

Soft faeces phase

Caecotrophs

Fig. 3. Overview of the activity of the digestive system in the rabbit. (*Adapted from* Harcourt-Brown F. Biologic characteristics of the domestic rabbit (*Oryctolagus cuniculi*). In: Harcourt-Brown F, editor. Textbook of Rabbit Medicine. Burlington (VT): Butterworth-Heinemann; 2002. p. 1–18; with permission.)

fermenters, further research on this condition is warranted. The diversity of bacterial flora and other organisms within the cecum is substantial, and includes many bacterial species dependent on location within the cecum lumen or wall; unidentified anaerobic species; ciliated and flagellate protozoa; and a rabbit-specific yeast.[8] *Lactobacillus* spp and *Escherichia coli* are usually absent from the normal gut flora of adult rabbits, but may be found in rabbits fed a high-carbohydrate, low-fiber diet.[1] Much remains to be learned and understood about the microbial populations of the rabbit hindgut and other herbivorous exotic companion mammal species. Fermentation produces volatile fatty acids, vitamins (B, C, and K), and proteins, which are eventually digested in the small intestine after cecotrophy. Cecotrophy occurs once or twice in a 24-hour period, usually at night. More than 74 strains of anaerobic bacteria have been isolated from the cecum mucosa of rabbits, and of those, very few have been identified.[10] The epithelium of the cecum has a high electrolyte transport capability suited to the large absorption of electrolytes.

In healthy and physically able rabbits, the large, soft, mucous-covered cecotrophs are ingested directly from the rectum (midnight snack) and swallowed whole. Multiple factors, including stimulation of rectal mechanoreceptors, perception of the cecotroph odor, and the blood concentrations of various metabolites and hormones, all stimulate the rabbit to directly ingest the cecotrophs. Higher-fiber diets increase cecophagy, whereas high-protein and low-fiber diets decrease cecophagy. Once eaten, the acidity of the stomach breaks down the protective mucous covering of the cecotroph. Continued digestion occurs in the small intestine, where cecotrophs represent an important component of the diet, providing protein, water, and vitamins.

In healthy rabbits on a high-fiber diet, the cecum contains a mixture of gram-positive bacilli, gram-negative bacteria (predominantly *Bacteroides* spp and some *E coli*), some yeasts, and protozoa. The usually stable synergistic microbial population in rabbits can be affected by a huge variety of internal and external factors, but 4 common factors encourage overgrowth of pathogens such as *Clostridium* spp and *E coli*:

1. Oral administration of inappropriate antibiotics can suppress the normal gram-positive flora and permit *Clostridia, E coli*, and other potentially pathogenic bacteria to flourish and predominate.
2. A diet low in fiber leads to low concentrations of fiber in the colon and cecum, which can result in the reduced production of VFA and an accompanying increase in pH, which destabilizes the microflora.
3. Inappropriate diets (low fiber, high carbohydrate) can lead to increased amounts of highly fermentable simple sugars in the cecum, which provide the major energy source for *Clostridial* overgrowth.
4. Excess dietary protein may cause an elevation of ammonia, the dissociation of which can alter cecal pH and cause dysbiosis.

Rabbits are naturally a prey animal; therefore, environmental stressors are also thought to act through the intermediary action of adrenaline or cortisol (probably on the fusus coli), causing ileus. Other environmental factors, including temperature, housing, and a variety of husbandry-related issues, can also have a significant impact on the microbial health of a rabbit's gastrointestinal system.

Colonic Separation Mechanisms

Coprophagy requires a digestive mechanism through which more valuable particles (mainly bacteria and small particles) are separated from less valuable components, such as indigestible or hardly digestible particulates. This mechanism has been termed a *colonic separation mechanism* (CSM).[11] The 2 primary mechanisms are the "wash-back" CSM found in lagomorphs and the "mucous-trap" CSM found in rodents.[12] CSMs are essential in coprophagic species for several reasons:

1. They ensure that protein synthesized by bacteria in the distal fermentation chambers, the cecum and colon, is not lost via defecation, but instead reingested along

with other bacterial products, such as vitamins or undigested remains of essential nutrients, such as fatty acids.[12]

2. The small body size of these species inhibits their ability to use body reserves to compensate for metabolic losses on low-quality forage, and therefore they need to maintain high food intake on low-quality forages and minimize metabolic losses via coprophagy.[13]

3. The species' reliance on microbiota to facilitate fermentation of plant structural carbohydrates. They need to retain a large percentage of this bacterial flora, because the bacterial multiplication time frame is longer than the food retention time.

4. Specific to the CSM of rabbits, minimizing the weight of their gut contents could be beneficial to minimizing body weight, and therefore enhancing their ability to run and evade predators.

The "wash-back" CSM separates fiber (based on size) and expels larger indigestible fibrous components from the body while retaining smaller components and fluid. This mechanism allows for the selective retention of fluids, bacteria, and smaller food components, which are effectively washed back into the cecum from the colon. This entire process is controlled by the fusus coli and culminates in the production of small, hard, dry fecal pellets from which water, electrolytes, and VFAs have been removed. Eventually larger, soft, mucous-covered cecotrophs are ingested directly from the anus.[11] This process/mechanism is essential in rabbits because they do not completely ferment fiber, and it is considered to be a more effective and efficient CSM than those of other species.

Rodents, such as guinea pigs and chinchillas, instead use a CSM referred to as the "mucous trap" CSM. These species have particular colonic anatomic feature, often referred to as the *colonic groove* or *furrow*, that is essential to the functionality of the mucous trap CSM. In this groove, mucous and bacteria are trapped and transported in a retrograde direction back to the cecum.[14,15] Guinea pigs and chinchillas are much more effective fermenters of fiber than rabbits, and therefore do not rely on the CSM to differentiate particulates of fiber. The "wash-back" CSM is characterized by short particle but long fluid retention times, whereas the "mucous trap" CSM results in a more or less simultaneous excretion of fluid and particle passage markers.[12]

The difference in soft feces produced by rabbits versus other rodents, such as guinea pigs and chinchillas, has been discussed and debated. In rabbits, the difference is evident between feces that are not reingested, commonly referred to as *hard feces*, and those that are reingested, referred as *cecotrophs* or *soft feces*,[16] whereas the visual difference between soft and hard feces in rodents is less evident.[17] Less identifiable cecotrophs in rodents is one of the reasons why the "wash-back" CSM of rabbits is considered more efficient than that of rodents.[17] Further evaluation of the key differences and functionalities of these CSMs is warranted.

GUINEA PIG

Guinea pigs (*Cavia porcellus*) are obligate herbivores and have a large tongue and narrow oral cavity. They have elodont teeth, which are open-rooted (constantly growing). Dental disease is a common malady, as discussed with rabbits, and proper diet (specifically ample fiber intake) is key to decreasing the likelihood of dental issues. Guinea pigs, like rabbits, are hindgut fermenters and coprophagic. Although the belief is that coprophagy is an important function in guinea pigs, its contribution to nutritional needs has not been fully characterized.[18] Coprophagy in rabbits is a key source of B vitamins and a means of optimizing the availability of proteins.[2] Guinea pigs, unlike rabbits, are not reliant on the key amount of B vitamins found in cecotrophs. Rabbits require a dietary source of 3 of the 10 B vitamins, whereas guinea pigs require a dietary source of 7.[19]

As discussed small herbivores use 1 of 2 primary CSMs necessary for coprophagy. This capability permits rapid passage of less-digestible food particles while retaining microorganisms, fluids, and more digestible food particles in the cecum to allow adequate opportunity for fermentation.[17] Rabbits use a multidirectional peristaltic motion (wash-back CSM) to separate components of fiber based on size, and mix these with other ingesta, bacteria, and water to concentrate more fermentable particles and eliminate larger particles of fiber. Guinea pigs and chinchillas use the "mucous-trap" CSM, in which bacteria from the cecum are trapped in the mucus of the colon with few to no food particles and returned to the colon through antiperistalsis.[18] The "mucous-trap" process is less efficient than the mechanisms used by rabbits.[12] Guinea pigs and chinchillas have a colonic furrow in the ascending colon, in which the concentration of bacteria and nitrogen is twice as high as in the lumen. This furrow allows for the transportation of bacteria from the proximal colon into the cecum as part of the separation mechanism.[18]

The stomach of guinea pigs contains the same 4 regions found in rabbits: the cardia, fundus, body, and pylorus. The stomach's inner surface is smooth and the pylorus consists of longitudinal folds or rugae. Unlike other rodents, the stomach of the guinea pig is completely glandular and does not contain a nonglandular portion.[20] The small intestine of guinea pigs is made up of 3 sections (duodenum, jejunum, and ileum), as found in most species. These sections are visually nondistinguishable, with the jejunum being the longest section ($\approx$ 90–100 cm). The cecum is the largest component of the guinea pig's gastrointestinal tract and contains upwards of 65% of the total contents.[21] The cecum has many lateral pouches (haustra) that are formed by the action of 3 taeniae coli (thick, longitudinal muscular bands that run the length of the large intestine).[18] The gastrointestinal flora is similar to that of the rabbit, being primarily grampositive, with anaerobic lactobacilli being the primary organisms in the large intestine.[2] As in the rabbit, a large number of additional organisms are prevalent, including yeast, protozoa, and other bacterial species. Gastric emptying time is approximately 2 hours and total gastrointestinal transit time is approximately 20 hours (8–30 hours), and considerably longer (up to 60 hours) if coprophagy is considered.[22]

CHINCHILLA

Chinchillas are obligate herbivores and hindgut fermenters, and cannot vomit. They are more similar to the guinea pig than the rabbit in terms of gastrointestinal anatomy, physiology, and CSM process. Their dentition is also more similar to that of guinea pigs than rabbits, because they have a larger grinding surface owing to a naturally higher-fiber and coarser diet than rabbits. They have elodont teeth, which are open-rooted (constantly growing). Chinchillas often have a yellow-orange color to their teeth, which is normal pigmentation. Chinchillas, like guinea pigs, differ from rabbits in that they have a palatal ostium (ie, an opening in the soft palate that connects the oropharynx and remainder of the pharynx). Compared with the guinea pig, the jejunum and descending colon of the chinchilla are long.[17] The colon is highly sacculated and the cecum large, yet the cecum holds fewer contents of the overall large intestine compared with rabbits and guinea pigs.[17] The cecum hold 23% of the dry matter content of the large intestine, compared with 57% in the rabbit and 44% in the guinea pig.[21]

Chinchillas, when compared with rabbits and guinea pigs, intensify their feed intake at night, with the highest activity occurring between 9:00 PM and 7:00 AM. They also show noticeable differences in rhythm of feed intake, palatability of individual ingredients, and capacity for digestion compared with rabbits and guinea pigs.[23]

NUTRITION

The discussion of the gastrointestinal system of herbivorous exotic companion mammals elucidates how integral proper diet is to the health of all small herbivores. The proper diet for small herbivores is provided in **Box 1 (Fig. 4)**.

High-quality, high-fiber grass hay should be available at all times. Although multiple varieties are available on the market, they have minimal nutritional difference, and therefore different species are appropriate, such as timothy, orchard, oat, meadow, and mixed, **(Table 1)**. Hay is a product of nature, and therefore will have variations in color, texture, feel, and taste. Because of this, it is important to transition between hay bags and offer different varieties of hay. Hay not only provides a key component of the nutritional needs of rabbits and other small herbivores but also encourages natural behaviors, such as foraging and grazing. Stimulating these natural behaviors may diminish boredom-based behaviors, increase foraging activity, and provide a sense of security to the animal.

Many commercially prepared diets are available to pet owners for purchase, the 2 most common being seed/cereal-based mixes and hay-based uniform pellets. Rabbits and other small herbivores are concentrate selectors and, if offered a mixed pellet, will select certain items from the mix, which will lead to improper and unbalanced nutrition. These mixes are often high in carbohydrates and simple sugars, which

---

Box 1
Components of a proper diet for small herivores

1. High-quality, high-fiber grass hay (approximately 70%–75%)
   a. Grass hay should be fed free-choice and available at all times. Any high-quality grass hay, such as timothy, orchard, meadow, or oat hay, is appropriate.
   b. These species will also use hay for bedding and nesting material. It is important to differentiate these different uses and ensure the animals always have access to clean fresh hay for ingestion.

2. High-fiber uniform pellets (approximately 15%–20%)
   a. These should be grass hay-, timothy-, or alfalfa-based, depending on life stage.
   b. Always feed only the recommended amount based on animal, age, weight, and health.
   c. It is important to avoid products that contain added seeds, fruits, or vegetables, or that use additional ingredients (typically starch- or carbohydrate-based) required for certain manufacturing techniques. These products not only allow for selective feeding behaviors but also are often nutritionally incomplete or unbalanced.

3. Fresh or dried greens (approximately 5%–15%)
   a. Only appropriate green plants should be fed, and all should be carefully cleaned. Organic products are preferred.
   b. Small amounts of appropriate vegetables and fruits are also beneficial.

4. Treats (approximately 0%–5%)
   a. Low-sugar, high-fiber treats are recommended.

5. Unlimited fresh, clean water
   a. Having more than one water source is always recommended, such as a bottle and crock.

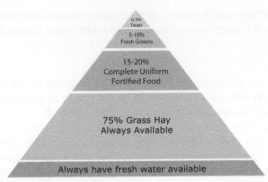

Fig. 4. Small herbivore feeding guidelines.

can lead to obesity and gastrointestinal problems. These mixes can also be low in fiber, which slows gastrointestinal motility and decreases normal dental wear. Uniform hay-based fortified pellets, high in fiber and low in protein, are recommended, because they eliminate selective feeding, thereby guaranteeing a proper vitamin and mineral intake.

Fresh greens are an important, necessary, and enjoyed component of a rabbit's and other small herbivore's diet. They provide an excellent source of water, enrichment, and additional nutrients, such as vitamins and minerals. Varying types and textures is a great enrichment tool. Washing all green completely is recommended, and organic products are preferable. A good in-depth reference of appropriate greens and vegetables can be found at http://rabbit.org/suggested-vegetables-and-fruits-for-a-rabbit-diet/.

Although treats are not required for rabbits or other small herbivores, limited appropriate treats can be beneficial for strengthening the pet/owner bond, training, and enrichment. It is important to limit the number of treats and ensure that they are low in protein, fat, calcium, and sugar. Some examples of inappropriate treats are nuts, seeds, popcorn, bread, crackers, and yogurt drops. High-fiber grass and alfalfa-based treats are appropriate, as are small amounts of freeze-dried fruits/veggies. Unfortunately, the marketplace is saturated with inappropriate and potential unhealthy treats, and therefore it is important for owners to understand which treats are healthy and which are not.

Table 1
Nutritional averages of commonly fed forages

Nutrient	Western Timothy Hay (%)	Orchard Grass Hay (%)	Oat Grass Hay (%)	Organic Meadow Grass (%)	Alfalfa Hay (%)
Crude protein	10.50–11.00	12.50–13.50	9.50–10.50	9.50–10.50	18.00–19.00
Crude fat	2.10–2.70	4.10–4.50	2.30–2.70	2.00–2.30	1.00–1.40
Crude fiber	24.80–26.50	24.10–26.00	26.90–27.90	24.00–25.90	17.10–19.50
Acid detergent fiber	29.00–30.50	27.00–28.50	29.00–30.30	29.00–30.40	27.00–28.40
Calcium	0.45	0.47	0.40	0.59	1.60
Phosphorus	0.22	0.28	0.22	0.18	0.27

WATER

Unlimited fresh, clean water is vital for small herbivores and should be available at all times. The water requirements of rabbits have been estimated at 50 to 100 mL/kg/d, depending on their diet.[24] Offering all exotic companion mammals water in more than one manner, such as in a sipper bottle and bowl/crock, is recommended to stimulate increased water intake. Actual water consumption can be significantly affected by diet and other environmental factors. Some species, such as guinea pigs, are prone to placing food material into the tip of water bottles when drinking, which can lead to potential blockage of the water bottle. Water should be changed daily, because bottles/bowls/crocks will become dirty from normal drinking.

SUMMARY

The gastrointestinal system of rabbits, guinea pigs, and chinchillas is complex and requires a high-fiber diet. Fiber is key to stimulating proper peristalsis, providing appropriate dental wear, and facilitating proper hindgut function, which leads to healthy microbial populations and cecotroph production. These animals are all concentrate selectors, hindgut fermenters, and coprophagic, and have open rooted dentition. They use unique CSMs—wash-back in rabbits and mucous-trap in guinea pigs/chinchillas—that allow them separate particles of food and bacteria based on importance to the system. Gastrointestinal disease is common in these species, and is often secondary to dietary or environmental factors.

REFERENCES

1. Harcourt-Brown F. Textbook of rabbit medicine. Boston: Butterworth-Heinemann; 2002.
2. Cheeke P. Rabbit feeding and nutrition. Orlando (FL): Academic Press; 1987.
3. Jenkins J. The veterinary clinics of North America. Exotic animal practice. Philadelphia: WB Saunders; 1999.
4. Alworth L, Harvey S. Chinchilla anatomy, physiology and behavior. In: Suckow M, Stevens K, Wilson R, editors. The laboratory rabbit, guinea pig, hamster and other rodents. London: Elsevier; 2012. p. 955–66.
5. Carabano R, Piquer J, Menoyo D, et al. The digestive system of the rabbit. In: de Blas C, Wiseman J, editors. Nutriton of the rabbit. 2nd edition. Cambridge (MA): CABI Publications; 2010. p. 1–18.
6. Wingerd B. Rabbit anatomy and dissection guide. Eden Prairie (MN): Blue Door Publishing; 2007.
7. Griffiths M, Davies D. The role of the soft pellets in the production of lactic acid in the rabbit stomach. J Nutr 1963;80:171–80.
8. Davies R, Davies J. Rabbit gastrointestinal physiology. Veterinary Clin North Am Exot Anim Pract 2003;6:139–53.
9. Snipes T, Clauss W, Weber A, et al. Structural and functional differences in various divisions of the rabbit colon. Cell Tissue Res 1982;225:331–46.
10. Straw T. Bacteria of the rabbit gut and their role in the health of the rabbit. Journal of Applied Rabbit Research 1988;11:142–6.
11. Bjornhag G. Comparative aspects of digestion in the hindgut of mammals. The colonic separation mechanism. Dtsch Tierarztl Wochenschr 1987;94:33–6.
12. Franz R, Kreuzer M, Hummel J, et al. Intake, selection, digesta retention, digestion and gut fill of two coprophageous species, rabbits (Orytolagus cuniculus) and guinea pigs (Cavia porcellus), on a hay only diet. J Anim Physiol Anim Nutr (Berl) 2010;95(5):564–70.
13. Meyer K, Hummel J, Clauss M. The relationship between forage cell wall content and voluntary food intake in mammalian herbivores. Mamm Rev 2010;40:221–45.

14. Tahahashi T, Sakaguchi E. Transport of bacteria across and along the large intestinal lumen of guinea pigs. J Comp Physiol 2006;176:173–8.
15. Holtenius K, Bjornhag G. The colonic separation mechanism I the guinea pig (Cavia porcellus) and the chinchilla (Chinchilla laniger). Comp Biochem Physiol 1985;82:537–42.
16. Hirakawa H. Coprophagy in leporids and other mammalian herbivores. Mamm Rev 2001;31:61–80.
17. Bjornhad G, Snipes R. Colonic separation mechanism in lagomorph and rodent species—a comparison. Zoosystematics and Evolution 1999;75:275–81.
18. Quesenberry K, Carpenter JW. Ferrets, rabbits, and rodents: clinical medicine and surgery. 3rd edition. St. Louis (MO): WB Saunders; 2012.
19. Stevens C, Hume I. Contributions of microbes in vertebrate gastrointestinal tract to production and conservation of nutrients. Physiol Rev 1998;78:393–427.
20. Harkness J, Murray K, Wagner J. Biology and diseases of guinea pigs. In: Fox J, Anderson L, Quimby F, editors. Laboratory animal medicine. 2nd edition. San Diego (CA): Academic Press; 2002. p. 203–46.
21. Hargaden M, Singer L. Guinea pig anatomy, physiology and behavior. In: Suckow M, Stevens K, Wilson R, editors. The laboratory rabbit, guinea pig, hamster and other rodents. London: Elsevier; 2012. p. 575–602.
22. Jilge B. The gastrointestinal transit time in the guinea pig. Z Versuchstierkd 1980; 22:204–10.
23. Wolf P, Schroder A, Wenger A, et al. Nutrition of the chinchilla as companion animal—data, influences and independences. J Anim Physiol Anim Nutr (Berl) 2003;87:129–33.
24. Brewer N, Cruise L. Physiology. In: Manning PJ, Ringler DH, Newcomer CE, et al, editors. The biology of the laboratory rabbit. 2nd edition. London: Academic Press; 1994. p. 63–70.

Diagnosis and Clinical Management of Gastrointestinal Conditions in Exotic Companion Mammals (Rabbits, Guinea Pigs, and Chinchillas)

Tracey K. Ritzman, DVM, DABVP (Avian & Exotic Companion Mammal)

KEYWORDS

- Gastroenterology • Exotic companion mammal • Rabbits • Guinea pigs
- Chinchillas • Ileus • Prokinetic therapy

KEY POINTS

- Presenting clinical signs of gastrointestinal disease in exotic companion mammals can vary widely.
- Small herbivores require specific dietary support and therapeutic treatments.
- Ileus is a common clinical condition and can be a primary or secondary disease.
- Common components of treatment of ileus include fluid therapy, pain relief, nutritional support, and prokinetic therapy.

INTRODUCTION

Presentation and clinical signs of gastrointestinal disease in exotic companion mammals are often nonspecific and varied. In this article, the diagnosis and clinical management (therapeutics) of gastrointestinal conditions in select exotic companion mammals are reviewed. The herbivore patient discussed includes rabbits, guinea pigs, and chinchillas.

Affected patients with gastrointestinal disorder may be asymptomatic, have nonspecific clinical changes, or may present with obvious abdominal complaints. A thorough physical examination should be performed on every exotic mammal patient as part of the medical evaluation. A detailed anamnesis aids the clinician in creating a differential diagnosis. The patient with gastrointestinal illness may have clinical signs such as change in character or frequency of stool production, change in appetite, tachypnea secondary to gastrointestinal enlargement or pain, change in posture or

Disclosure: This article originally appeared in similar form in the proceedings of the 2013 Association of Exotic Mammal Veterinarians Conference in Indianapolis, Indiana, USA.
Cascade Hospital for Animals, 6730 Cascade Road Southeast, Grand Rapids, MI 49546, USA
E-mail address: tritzman@chfa.net

activity, bruxism, vomiting (some species), diarrhea, melena, or general malaise. Diarrhea should be characterized as acute or chronic, and if possible, as small bowel or large bowel in origin. Large bowel diarrhea is often characterized by increased mucus or frank blood in the stool. Dental disease should be considered in patients having difficulty prehending or chewing food, displaying a change in dietary preferences, or showing a generalized decreased appetite.

DIAGNOSIS OF GASTROINTESTINAL DISEASE

A presumptive diagnosis of gastrointestinal disease can often be obtained from the history, physical examination, and initial diagnostics. Differential diagnoses for a gastrointestinal condition depend on the species, symptoms, and diagnostic findings. Noninvasive and often initial diagnostics that can be used for the diagnosis of gastrointestinal disease include hematology, chemistry and electrolyte testing, blood gas analysis, imaging (radiography or ultrasonography), fecal parasite testing, fecal direct, fecal Gram stain, or fecal bacterial culture and sensitivity testing.

Sedation or brief general anesthesia is often necessary in the exotic companion mammal patient for the clinician to safely and efficiently perform a thorough oral examination. Sedation or brief general anesthesia may also be necessary to obtain blood samples and diagnostic quality imaging. More advanced testing for the diagnosis of gastrointestinal conditions in small mammals can include endoscopic examination of the oral cavity to evaluate the teeth and soft tissues of the mouth, esophagus, stomach, or proximal small intestinal tract. Other diagnostic options, which are more invasive, include endoscopic biopsies, surgical exploration and evaluation, or surgical biopsies of the gastrointestinal system or associated internal organs (liver, gallbladder, pancreas). Asymptomatic lesions may be discovered incidentally during survey radiography or during other abdominal imaging studies, such as ultrasonography.

Imaging is an essential diagnostic tool for the veterinary clinician working with exotic companion mammals. With the advancement of imaging and the availability of digital radiography systems, the detail obtained can be excellent. Imaging options available for exotic companion mammals include radiography, ultrasonography, computed tomography (CT), or magnetic resonance imaging (MRI). Initial imaging usually includes radiography or ultrasonography, because CT and MRI are inherently more expensive tests and are not available at most veterinary clinics. For initial assessment, whole-body ventrodorsal and lateral views should be taken to allow for evaluation of the entire thorax and abdomen, including liver, gastrointestinal tract, reproductive organs, and urinary system. If dental disease is suspected, skull or dental radiographs may also be indicated. Cost and accessibility of the more sophisticated imaging options may be limiting factors with veterinary patients.

For all species discussed in this article, the stomach is normally located in the left cranial quadrant of the abdomen. With imaging, the size, positioning, and contents of the stomach should be evaluated. The intestinal tract can be examined for luminal size, position within the abdomen, wall thickness, and pattern. If dilation or plication is noticed within the intestinal tract, the clinician should consider obstruction or foreign body disease in the differential for the patient. Intestinal obstructive disease may lead to dilation of the intestine proximal to the obstruction. With obstructive disease, the loops of bowel are often greater than twice the width of lumbar vertebrae number 2 (L2) on imaging.[1] Gastric outflow obstruction may be indicated with imaging if the stomach is distended. Because rabbits, guinea pigs, and chinchillas are unable to vomit, gastric dilation can occur rapidly. Gastric dilation and torsion have been documented in guinea pigs.[2] Torsion of the root of the mesentery can also occur in guinea pigs.[2] Liver torsion has been diagnosed in rabbits with radiography and ultrasonography imaging.[2] Abnormal positioning of the stomach on the right side of the body or caudal to the small intestinal loops is cause for concern and potential surgical intervention. The application and usefulness of ultrasonography for herbivore mammals can be limited, because of interference from the normal presence of gas within the cecum/large intestinal tract (**Figs. 1** and **2**).

With most gastrointestinal conditions, hematology results are often nonspecific, and may not reflect specific changes related to the primary disease. Baseline blood work including a complete blood cell count and biochemistry profile is a starting point for diagnostic evaluation of the exotic companion mammal patient. These tests allow the clinician to evaluate for systemic change and organ function. Chronic inflammatory conditions such as gastrointestinal infection or inflammatory bowel disease may show a mild to moderate lymphocytosis. Anemia, panleukopenia, or thrombocytopenia may be noted if there is blood lost from the gastrointestinal tract (ulceration, perforation) or bone marrow involvement with a disease syndrome. Patients with gastrointestinal neoplasia such as lymphoma can either have unremarkable blood work or may have changes in the white blood cell count and differential consistent with a leukocytosis, often with a lymphocytosis. A leukocytosis greater than 20,000/uL may be associated with lymphoid neoplasia, often lymphoma. The biochemistry profile with gastrointestinal disease may be normal or may reflect changes associated with blood protein levels or hepatic or pancreatic function.

The presence of an abnormal soft tissue mass effect involving the gastrointestinal system can lead to disruption of normal function. Neoplasia is a concern if single or multiple abnormal soft tissue masses or organomegaly are evident on imaging. As with most neoplasms, hematology results are often nonspecific and may not reflect specific changes related to the primary disease. A definitive diagnosis of neoplasia requires a histopathologic evaluation of a representative tissue sample from the mass or affected organ. Cytologic evaluation of the feces may aid in the diagnosis of certain conditions such as bacterial gastroenteritis or parasitic disease. Examination of the feces for intestinal parasites is indicated for most species if stool is abnormal. Fecal screening tests used for canine and feline patients can be applied to exotic mammals. Fecal bacterial culture testing can be useful in some cases or for routine health screening. Urine testing is possible for exotic mammals. To decrease the risk of iatrogenic bladder injury or rupture, cystocentesis is often preferred over manual expression of the bladder. Sedation or anesthesia helps to reduce the risk of injury to the

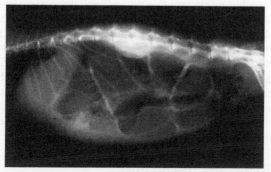

Fig. 1. Right lateral abdominal radiograph of adult pet rabbit with severe gas distention of the cecum. The haustra of the cecum are clearly visible, indicating that the enlarged structure is the cecum.

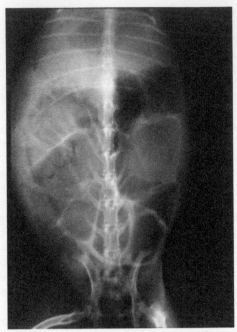

Fig. 2. Ventrodorsal abdominal radiograph of adult pet rabbit with severe gas distention of the cecum. The haustra of the cecum are clearly visible, indicating that the enlarged structure is the cecum.

patient or the bladder when performing cystocentesis. In the literature, repetitive puncture of the bladder has been implicated as a factor with calculus formation.[3] Depending on patient size, urinary catheterization can be performed in anesthetized patients for urine sample collection or flushing of the bladder.

Surgical diagnostics, although invasive, can often provide a definitive diagnosis through direct visual examination of the internal organs and with collection of tissue biopsies and histopathology. Endoscopy can be used in some of the larger species of exotic companion mammals such as rabbits and ferrets, but the small size of many of the rodent species often limits the use of this diagnostic modality.

There are many different ways to perform anesthesia in exotic companion mammals, and recommended drugs and dosing vary and depend on the species.[4,5]

Critically ill patients should be stabilized before consideration of sedation or anesthesia. Intubation for respiratory support should be performed when possible. Rabbits greater than 1.36 kg (3 lb) body weight can often be intubated.[4,5] Histopathology is an essential diagnostic tool for a definitive diagnosis of some conditions. It is recommended for the clinician to use a board-certified veterinary pathologist with knowledge and experience of exotic mammal tissues when submitting samples. Good perioperative care for patient support during and after surgery includes the use of an effective pain management protocol, fluid support, body temperature regulation with thermal support, and a quiet recovery area.

CLINICAL MANAGEMENT AND THERAPEUTICS

Clinical management and therapeutics for gastrointestinal disease vary based on the specific diagnosis. Some key therapeutic points for the management of the small herbivores include basing the treatment plan on the specific gastrointestinal condition diagnosed. For true gastrointestinal obstructive disease, surgical treatment is required. For nonsurgical conditions, the treatment plan is based on the diagnosis, patient condition at the time of diagnosis, the species, and anatomy and physiology of the patient.

The most common components of medical therapy for nonsurgical gastrointestinal conditions include fluid therapy, pain management, nutritional support, medication to help promote normal gastrointestinal function and motility and, in rare cases if indicated, antimicrobial therapy.[6–18] Antiparasitic therapy would be provided for patients with indication of parasitic disease. Gastric ulcers have the potential to occur in these species. Gastrointestinal protectants should be considered as part of the treatment plan when indicated.

The Hospital Setting

For the in-hospital patient receiving treatment, the cage or incubator should be appropriate for the size of the patient and it should be located in a quiet area. It is best to house rabbits, guinea pigs, and chinchillas in a separate area of the hospital and away from predator species. The staff handling and treating these patients should have training in how to safely and effectively handle and treat, minimizing patient stress. Unless contraindicated, appropriate foods should be available at all times for herbivores, including fresh grass hays, fresh vegetables, and some pellets.

Administration of medication can be challenging for small mammals. In the hospital setting, the clinician may choose to give some medications in injectable form. Subcutaneous injections are well tolerated by most species and are suitable for most parenteral medications, with the exception of some anesthetic agents. Some clients are even able to learn and administer subcutaneous injections at home. Oral medications are most often given at home. Most pills need to be compounded into a flavored liquid suspension for use with rabbits, guinea pigs, and chinchillas. A compounding pharmacy can be a great resource for the clinician when considering how to prescribe and administer medications.

Fluid Therapy

Fluid therapy is a core component in the treatment of gastrointestinal conditions in almost all patients. Route of administration can include the intravenous, intraosseous, subcutaneous, or oral route. The intravenous route is the most effective and is the preferred route for debilitated patients. For each patient, it is important for the clinician to evaluate the need for intravenous access. The potential stress involved with placement and maintenance of an intravenous catheter must be weighed against the clinical benefit of this form of treatment. Unless severely debilitated, most exotic mammal patients can tolerate placement of an intravenous catheter. Occasionally, sedation or brief general anesthesia may be required for catheter placement. Sites most often used for intravenous catheter placement in rabbits include the cephalic or lateral saphenous veins. A 24-gauge or 26-gauge catheter can be used in smaller rabbits. For rabbits weighing more than 2.26 kg (5 lb), a 22-gauge catheter can often be used. Although the marginal ear vein is a potential site for intravenous catheter placement in the rabbit, it is not recommended to use this site for pet animals, because of the potential for tissue necrosis and sloughing of the tip of the pinna. From an aesthetic standpoint, this factor can be an issue with clients. However, the marginal ear vein is used in some laboratory research settings with rabbits.

The cephalic or saphenous vein is most often used in guinea pigs and chinchilla patients. If the patient is too small or has too much peripheral vasoconstriction to allow for intravenous access, an intraosseous catheter route is a good option for most exotic mammals. Placement of an intraosseous catheter requires analgesia and brief anesthesia for placement. Sites for intraosseous catheter placement include the greater trochanter of the femur, the tibial crest, or the proximal humerus. A spinal needle or intraosseous catheter can be used as an intraosseous catheter. The size depends on the patient and is usually 18-gauge to 22-gauge and 2.54 to 3.81 cm (1–1.5 in) long. Most exotic mammal patients tolerate an indwelling catheter if the associated discomfort is minimized with good pain management. Elizabethan collars are stressful to exotic mammal patients and may prevent normal cecotrophy and food intake. Their use should be avoided when possible. Maintenance fluid therapy is estimated to be 50 to 70 mL/kg/24 h for the rabbit patient, and approximately 60 mL/kg/24 h in the guinea pig and chinchilla patient.[6] Healthy rabbits normally consume approximately 100 to 150 mL/kg/d of water.[6] Even if dehydration is not obvious, with gastrointestinal disorders, there is often a fluid deficit or imbalance in the patient. Two times maintenance therapy is recommended for these patients, if it can be tolerated. Patients with known cardiac disease or other disorders may require a more conservative rate of fluid administration. It is best to use infusion fluid pumps with exotic mammals to regulate fluid delivery and minimize the risk of accidental fluid overload (**Fig. 3**).

Subcutaneous fluid therapy can be given either into the scruff of the neck in the interscapular region or the loose skin over the chest. Usually, the more dorsal location is preferred to help reduce the risk of dependent edema. With subcutaneous fluid treatment, the dosage can vary but is often in the range of 100 to 120 mL/kg/d divided into several treatments throughout the day (2 or 3 times daily). In general, 20 to 40 mL/kg can be given subcutaneously in 1 location.[6]

Rarely are medications given intramuscularly to exotic mammals. This caveat is in part because of their small body size and limited muscle mass. If a medication has to be given intramuscularly, it is best to divide large volumes (>0.5 mL/kg) into several sites. There is potential for tissue damage or muscle necrosis with any intramuscular injection. For this reason, care should be taken if this route is chosen, and the number of injections should be minimized.

Intravenous injections for single injection can be given in the peripheral leg vein (cephalic or saphenous vein) of most species. The small patient size and short length of the limbs of many of these patients can make intravenous injections challenging. It is best to have an indwelling intravenous catheter placed if repeated intravenous

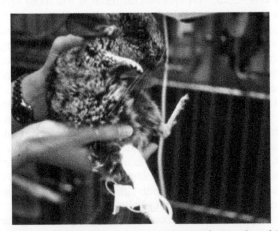

Fig. 3. Chinchilla patient with a peripheral intravenous catheter placed in the right lateral saphenous vein for fluid therapy.

injections are required for treatment. The ear vein is not a preferred site for use in rabbits for intravenous injections, because of the potential for tissue sloughing, as mentioned earlier.

Vascular access ports are another option to use in exotic companion mammals for patients requiring repeated intravenous access. I used a vascular access port in a chinchilla patient to allow for intravenous access for chemotherapy.[19] Vascular access ports consist of a titanium port, which is placed surgically in the subcutaneous tissue, as well as sterile tubing, which is surgically fed into the desired adjacent blood vessel. The vascular access port can then be used with special needles for blood sample collection or repeated injections, minimizing the risk of extravascular complications.

Pain Management

Pain management is an essential component of treatment of a successful outcome for the exotic mammal patient. Many gastrointestinal conditions can lead to significant pain and discomfort for the patient. Gas distention or impaction of the stomach or intestinal tract can make a patient uncomfortable and less likely to eat. Multimodal pain relief is an ideal option, if available and appropriate for the patient. Both medical and surgical conditions require good pain control. Use of both an analgesic (such as buprenorphine or butorphanol) combined with a nonsteroidal antiinflammatory (such as meloxicam) can be effective at reducing discomfort, reducing inflammation, and promoting a positive outcome.[20] The duration of action of pain relief medications varies widely depending on species and the class of medication.[20] In general, for exotic mammals, nonsteroidal antiinflammatory medications are estimated to be effective for a longer period than opioid drugs. The recommended dosage for pain relief medication varies depending on the drug and the target species. The veterinary clinician is advised to consult an up-to-date exotics formulary for specific dosage recommendations for each species.[21,22]

Opioids are some of the most effective analgesics available for the systemic treatment of acute pain in many species, including exotic companion mammals. Opioids are used extensively to provide analgesia and, sometimes, anesthesia. Opioids combine reversibly with specific receptors in the brain, spinal cord, and periphery, altering the transmission and perception of pain. In addition to analgesia, opioids can induce other central nervous system (CNS) effects, including sedation, euphoria, dysphoria, and excitement.[4,5,20] The clinical effects of opioids vary between the μ opioid receptor agonists (ie, morphine, hydromorphone), partial μ agonists (ie, buprenorphine), and agonist-antagonists (ie, butorphanol). Species and individual differences in the response to opioids are marked, requiring the careful selection of opioid and adjustment of dose for different species.[4,5,20] The most frequently used opioids for rabbits, guinea pigs, and chinchillas include buprenorphine and butorphanol.[4,5,20] Potential side effects of opioids in rabbits, guinea pigs, and chinchillas include respiratory or mental depression, hypothermia, and bradycardia.[4,5,20] Although there is potential for opioids to affect gastrointestinal motility, this is infrequently noted with use in most exotic mammal patients.

Nonsteroidal antiinflammatory drugs (NSAIDs) are useful medications in the treatment of postsurgical pain in a variety of species.[4,5,20,23,24] Decreasing inflammation after surgery or trauma can greatly improve analgesia. Inflammation is a key component in both peripheral and central sensitization leading to pain. Significant advantages of NSAID therapy include wide availability, a relatively long duration of action, low cost, and ease of administration.[23,24] NSAIDs have long been used to decrease inflammation and provide analgesia. NSAID therapy can be considered as part of the analgesic plan if the animal does not have preexisting renal, hepatic, coagulation, or ulcer-related gastrointestinal problems. NSAIDs should be administered only to well-hydrated patients. Meloxicam is a specific NSAID often used in exotic mammal species such as rabbits, guinea pigs, and chinchillas.[4,5,20,23,24] Meloxicam can be used postoperatively in the stable and hydrated small mammal patient when they start eating.

Renal values should ideally be checked before prescribing NSAIDs. It is not recommended to use NSAIDs as a preanesthetic drug in the critically ill patient. Administration of meloxicam before general anesthesia is controversial, because of the risk of hypotension in some patients under anesthesia.[23,24]

Tramadol, an increasingly popular veterinary drug for pain relief in veterinary patients, is a centrally acting agent with multimodal analgesic effects. Tramadol may be used alone to treat mild pain or combined with other types of pain relief medications in a multimodal plan for treating moderate to severe pain.[4,5,21] Tramadol has moderate affinity for the μ opioid receptor. It also inhibits neuronal uptake of norepinephrine and serotonin, monoamine neurotransmitters involved in descending inhibitory pathways in the CNS.[4,5,20] Compared with pure μ agonists, tramadol results in less sedation, less respiratory depression, and improved oral bioavailability. It also has the advantage of not being a controlled substance. Possible side effects include decreased seizure thresholds, nausea/vomiting, and in some animals, altered behavior. There are few clinical studies examining the use of tramadol in veterinary species.

In rabbits, there have been limited pharmacokinetic studies to evaluate plasma levels after administration of tramadol.[25] Caution is warranted in patients receiving monoamine oxidase inhibitors or selective serotonin (5-hydroxytryptamine) reuptake inhibitors, because of the increased risk of serotonin syndrome.[25]

Corticosteroids such as dexamethasone, prednisone, and prednisolone are drugs that reduce inflammation and provide analgesia. Corticosteroids are used less frequently in the postoperative period, because of the potential for decreasing immune function and other well-known side effects (ie, polyphagia, polydipsia, polyuria) after repeated dosing. Corticosteroid and NSAID therapy should not be administered concurrently. Corticosteroid treatment is commonly used in canine and feline patients for treatment of various inflammatory and pain conditions. With exotic companion mammals, corticosteroids should be used judiciously because of the potential side effects, particularly the impact on immune function. Many rabbit, guinea pig, and chinchilla patients have potential occult systemic bacterial disease (ie, *Pasteurella* infection), which could flare with immune suppression.

Nutritional Support

Maintaining a positive energy balance and gastrointestinal function for hospitalized exotic mammals is crucial for a good clinical outcome, regardless of the original cause of illness. As with any patient recovering from illness, it is important to meet nutritional and fluid needs during treatment. A comprehensive treatment plan should include steps for meeting nutritional goals. Providing for the increased or unique dietary needs of a patient during illness and surgical recovery presents an even greater challenge than just meeting daily nutritional requirements. Animals that are ill or debilitated from disease often present anorexic. Even if the original illness was not nutritional in origin, secondary changes from anorexia can quickly develop. These secondary physiologic complications can lead to increased morbidity or mortality. The logistics alone of providing nutritional support to an anorexic exotic mammal patient is a challenge even to the most astute clinician.

An estimate of the daily energy requirement can be made for the debilitated small herbivore patient using the formula MER (metabolizable energy requirement) = 250 × (wt [kg])$^{0.75}$.

It is imperative for the patient to keep a positive energy balance to prevent secondary hepatic lipidosis, which can develop quickly as a result of gastrointestinal disease or surgery. The mechanisms involved for inducing hepatic lipidosis are not completely known. Possible causes include protein deficiency, excessive peripheral lipolysis, excessive lipogenesis, inhibition of synthesis, and secretion of very low-density lipoproteins, and inhibition of lipid oxidation. Ketosis can also develop rapidly in some herbivore patients who are not eating well on their own. Ketosis occurs as the result of increased energy demand accompanied by insufficient nutrition. This condition can occur in pregnant herbivores and can be related to stress during pregnancy, fasting, improper nutrition (fiber too low), and can be associated with pregnancy toxemia.

Assisted feeding via the enteral route

If you must assist the patient with feeding, it is optimal to use the enteral route for nutritional support when possible. This route simulates the natural route of feeding and promotes return to normal gastrointestinal function by using the gastrointestinal tract directly.

Options for assist feeding via the enteral route include making a homemade syringe-feeding mixture or using a commercially available prepared syringe food appropriate for herbivores. A homemade feeding gruel can be made by pulverizing pellets into a fine powder mixed either with baby food (apple or carrot baby food works best) or canned pumpkin. A small pinch of powdered *Lactobacillus acidophilus* can be added to the mixture. Several commercial gruel foods for herbivores are available that can be effective. These products are a hay-based syringe-feeding formula that is mixed with water to produce a high-fiber mixture for anorectic herbivores. These products have been developed to provide adequate fiber and other nutrient levels and are still fine enough to use with a feeding syringe. Also available commercially is a finer-consistency tube-feeding product that allows for use in feeding tubes. This option reduces the risk of occlusion of the feeding tube with fibrous material, which often occurs with homemade gruel diets (**Fig. 4**).

The product being fed should be mixed well to a liquid consistency. The gruel should be mixed fresh at each feeding to prevent spoilage. The patient is fed in a sternal position. For rabbits and other small herbivores, it is often helpful to wrap the patient in a towel to aid in restraint and prevent struggle. Gently open the mouth and insert the syringe at the diastema (the gap between the front incisors and cheek teeth) and administer slowly, taking great care to avoid aspiration. Although this feeding method

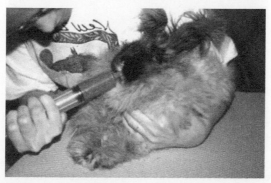

Fig. 4. Angora rabbit being syringe fed an enteral herbivore gruel for nutritional support.

can be time consuming, it can be an effective way to deliver the formula and is noninvasive to the patient. Give the rabbit plenty of time to swallow between servings. For rabbits, usually 3 to 4 feedings of approximately 10 to 15 mL per feeding cause the gastrointestinal tract to move again. Smaller herbivores require a smaller volume for the feeding amount. Fresh greens are often successful in getting a rabbit to eat again on its own. Cilantro and parsley are often favorites for rabbits, and offerings of these fresh herbs can often entice rabbit patients to eat (**Fig. 5**).

Make sure that all hay is fresh, free of dust or mold spores, and does not harbor any thorns or foreign objects, such as sticks, pieces of plants, or thistles. Fresh hay should be green, soft or silky to the touch, and have a fresh aroma. Hay should not be used if it is wet or appears to be dusty, dirty, moldy, or old. Hay is best purchased in small bales packaged for small herbivores rather than using a horse-sized bale.

Rabbits drink a large volume of water for their body size, so provide adequate, clean water at all times. Clean and inspect water systems daily, because many rabbits chew on the ends of the sipper straw and damage it. Clean and disinfect the water bowls daily, because they are easily contaminated.

Orogastric tube feeding

Orogastric tubes can be used for single dosing for nutritional support. This method of providing nutrition is not considered acceptable for long-term or chronic nutritional support. Depending on the demeanor and size of the patient, orogastric tube feeding may not be possible. Larger rabbits can accommodate an orogastric tube, whereas smaller patients may not be large enough for passage of the tube down the esophagus. This method of feeding is most often used for rabbit patients rather than for smaller herbivore species.

For orogastric tube feeding, one should premeasure the length of tube needed from the mouth to the level of the last rib, where the stomach would be located. A mouth gag is required to prevent the patient from biting down on the tube, which could sever the tube. For feeding, an 18-French to 22-French round tube rubber catheter is used. The tube is gently passed down the esophagus to the stomach. Placement is checked and verified to be in the stomach before administration of food material. This check is important to reduce the risk of aspiration. Placement can be verified with radiograph imaging. Another way to check tube placement is to push a small amount of air can through the tube while auscultating at the level of stomach. Checking for negative pressure when the tube is backed into the esophagus can also assess proper

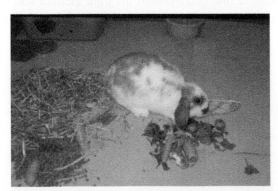

Fig. 5. A lop-eared rabbit patient that is in hospital being treated for ileus. Note the large selection of food items placed in the hospital cage to entice the rabbit to eat. Foods include fresh vegetables and produce, plenty of grass hay, and a limited amount of pellets.

placement of the tube. For many patients, light sedation may be required for this procedure, because it can be stressful to the patient.

Nasogastric tube feeding

Nasogastric tubes are used with exotic companion mammal patients for sustained nutritional support. One challenge of using this method is that the continuous presence of the nasogastric tube can be stressful to the patient. Many rabbits and other species of small herbivores do not tolerate a nasogastric tube well. The length of tube required is measured as described for orogastric tube placement. For nasogastric tubes, a smaller tube diameter is required to pass through the nasal passage. A pediatric feeding tube size 3.5 to 5 French can be used for most rabbits. Light sedation may be required for tube placement, depending on patient demeanor and condition. A topical anesthetic such as 2% lidocaine gel or several drops of proparacaine (Ophthaine, Solvay Animal Health, Medora Heights, MN) can be placed in the nasal opening before tube placement. The tube is gently inserted through the ventromedial nasal meatus and passed ventrally and medially while the patient's head is flexed. Proper placement of the nasogastric tube is confirmed with radiographic imaging. The tube is secured in place by using a small amount of cyanoacrylate glue on the dorsal nasal area or suturing of the tube with a tape tab to the top of the head. Occasionally, an Elizabethan collar may be required to prevent the patient from scratching or removing the tube. Removal can usually be performed without the need for sedation. Disadvantages of this feeding method include stress to the patient and the need to use a finer grind powder to prevent clogging of the tube.

Parenteral nutrition

Parenteral nutrition (PN) has been used successfully in canine and feline patients but is infrequently discussed in regards to exotic companion mammal patients. In my experience, this form of nutritional support can be used safely and effectively in rabbits and ferrets. The basis for providing PN to exotic mammals is similar to the parameters used for dogs and cats.[26] There are different levels of protein intake based on the patient's primary nutritional classification (eg, herbivore vs carnivore).[26] A PN solution can adequately meet the resting energy requirement (RER) and most, but not all, of the essential amino, fatty acids, water soluble vitamins, and some macro and trace minerals for exotic mammals.[26]

When using a PN solution, it is important to have it compounded by a reputable veterinary nutrition service. All-in-one PN bags can be purchased from several sources.[26] Some veterinary schools, large referral hospitals, or a veterinary nutritional specialist can serve as resources for the general practitioner. The PN solution should provide an energy source that should meet, but ideally not exceed by much, the RER for the patient.[26] Excess caloric intake to small mammal patients can result in metabolic complications.

The PN solution can be delivered to the patient via a central, peripheral, intraosseous, or intraperitoneal catheter. The osmolarity of the solution dictates the route that can be used. PN solutions with osmolarity of greater than 550 mOsm/L should be given through a central vein.[26] A peripheral vein can be used for PN solutions of lower osmolarity (<550 mOsm/L) (**Fig. 6**).[26]

Potential side effects of PN use in the exotic mammal include the potential for catheter complications, which can include potential thrombophlebitis or infection.[26] Infection complications are usually related to substandard catheter care rather than a problem with the PN solution. An aseptic technique must be followed with placement and maintenance of intravenous catheters used for PN therapy. For therapy longer

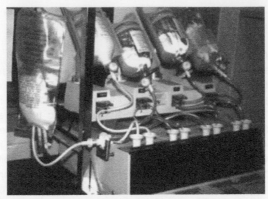

Fig. 6. PN mixing machine. The nutritionist determines the nutrient components required for a specific patient. This information is entered and the machine creates the sterile mixture with the appropriate ratio of nutrients.

than 3 days, it is best to use polyurethane or silicone catheters.[26] Expense can also be a factor with PN, because the cost of this form of therapy is considerably higher than using the enteral route. This expense is in part a result of the need for hospitalization and catheter maintenance during the treatment period for PN therapy.

Monitoring of Gastrointestinal Function and Response During Treatment

Regardless of the route of nutritional support used for the patient, the veterinary clinician should have some basic parameters to use for gauging patient progress. Depending on species, these clinical signs can be used to help the veterinary staff and clients determine if their patient is making positive progress with treatment.

A healthy exotic mammal should be passing urine and fecal material in a normal manner. The appearance, consistency, and frequency should be noted. What is normal for a patient varies depending on size, species, and route of nutrition.

Positive clinical signs to watch for herbivores include round, formed, hard droppings being produced in moderate to large amounts. Urine should be clear or yellow. In rabbits, urine changes color frequently, depending on calcium content and the amount of normal pigments present in the urine. Moist, grapelike clusters of cecotrophs should be produced and ingested by the rabbit patient (**Fig. 7**).

Potential negative clinical signs to look for when monitoring response to nutritional therapy include lack of stool production, soft, runny, or sludgy piles of stool, excessive

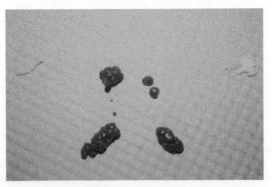

Fig. 7. Normal cecotrophs from a rabbit.

fibers or mucus holding droppings together, or excess mucus in stool. Real blood clots in urine or stool are also a concern. Lack of urine production or fecal droppings over a 24-hour period warrants evaluation of clinical progress and condition. Visible parasites in the stool are also a concern.

Clinical signs for clients to monitor at home with their pets can include diminished appetite, lack of fecal dropping, diarrhea, unusual stool formation or blood/mucus in the stool, sloshing sounds in the abdomen, swelling and soreness in the abdominal area, unusual enlargements, wet tail (diarrhea that causes complications at the peri-neal area), prolapsed bowel, unexplained weight loss, limited movement, and loss of appetite. Clients who notice any of these symptoms at home should have their pet examined by a veterinary clinician as soon as possible.

Prokinetic Therapy

The use of prokinetic medication can be beneficial for patients experiencing hypomo-tility of the gastrointestinal tract. This class of medication helps to promote normal gastrointestinal motility and function in nonobstructed patients. The use of prokinetic medication is contraindicated in patients with potential or known obstructive disease. Prokinetics can be used with the medical treatment of ileus or preoperatively and post-operatively for patients undergoing surgery. Dosing information can be obtained in published studies for these species.[21,22] Prokinetic medications frequently used in rabbits, guinea pigs, and chinchillas include metoclopramide, cisapride, and ranitidine.[4,5,11–13,18]

Metoclopramide is a dopaminergic antagonist and peripheral serotonin receptor antagonist with gastrointestinal and CNS effects.[11,13,21] In the upper gastrointestinal tract, metoclopramide increases both acetylcholine release from neurons and cholin-ergic receptor sensitivity to acetylcholine.[21] Metoclopramide stimulates and coordi-nates esophageal, gastric, pyloric, and duodenal motor activity. It increases lower esophageal sphincter tone and stimulates gastric contractions and relaxes the pylorus and duodenum.[21] Inadequate cholinergic activity is implicated in many gastrointes-tinal motility disorders; therefore, metoclopramide should be most effective in dis-eases in which normal motility is diminished or impaired. Metoclopramide speeds gastric emptying of liquids, but may slow the emptying of solids. It is effective in treat-ing postoperative ileus in exotic mammals, which is often characterized by decreased gastrointestinal activity and motility. Metoclopramide has little or no effect on the distal gastrointestinal tract (colonic motility). Metoclopramide readily crosses the blood-brain barrier, where dopamine antagonism at the chemoreceptor trigger zone produces an antiemetic effect.[21] However, dopamine antagonism in the striatum causes adverse effects known collectively as extrapyramidal signs, which include involuntary muscle spasms, motor restlessness, and inappropriate aggression.[21] These adverse effects are more commonly noted in humans than in veterinary patients.

Cisapride is chemically related to metoclopramide, but unlike metoclopramide, it does not cross the blood-brain barrier or have antidopaminergic effects.[21] Therefore, it does not have antiemetic action or cause extrapyramidal effects (extreme CNS stimulation).[21] Cisapride enhances the release of acetylcholine from postganglionic nerve endings of the myenteric plexus and antagonizes the inhibitory action of sero-tonin on the myenteric plexus, resulting in increased gastrointestinal motility and heart rate.[21] Cisapride is more potent and has broader prokinetic activity than meto-clopramide, increasing the motility of the colon, as well as that of the esophagus, stomach, and small intestine.[21] Cisapride can be useful in preventing postoperative ileus in exotic companion mammals.[4,5,11–13,18] Cisapride for animal patients can be obtained only through compounding veterinary pharmacies because the manufacturer voluntarily placed it under a limited-access program as a result of human side effects. In humans, cases of heart rhythm disorders and deaths were reported to the US Food and Drug Administration. These cardiac problems in humans were highly associated with concurrent drug therapy or specific underlying conditions. In veterinary medicine, adverse reactions to clinical use of cisapride have not generally been reported.

Ranitidine is a histamine H_2-receptor antagonist, which is a prokinetic as well as an inhibitor of gastric acid secretion.[21] The prokinetic activity is caused by acetylcholinesterase inhibition, with the greatest activity in the proximal gastrointestinal tract.[21] Ranitidine stimulates gastrointestinal motility by increasing the amount of acetylcholinesterase available to bind to smooth muscle muscarinic receptors.[21] It also stimulates colonic smooth muscle contractions through a cholinergic mechanism. Ranitidine has the added benefit of reducing gastric ulceration through the inhibition of gastric acid secretion.[21]

Antibiotic Therapy

Antibiotic therapy should be used only if truly indicated. Rabbits, guinea pigs, and chinchillas have a delicate gastrointestinal system in terms of microbial flora. Normal gastrointestinal bacterial flora for these species is mostly gram-positive bacteria and anaerobes. The use of antibiotics that suppress the normal flora can result in the overgrowth of pathogenic organisms. The use of antibiotics with a gram-positive spectrum should be avoided. Failure to follow this advice could lead to antibiotic-induced dysbiosis. Dysbiosis can cause severe diarrhea, enterotoxemia, severe fluid loss, and even death. Antibiotics to avoid include the β-lactams (cephalosporins and oral penicillin) and the macrolides (lincomycin, clindamycin, erythromycin). Parenteral penicillin (injectable form) is safe to use in rabbits subcutaneously but should not be given orally, because of risk of dysbiosis.

THERAPEUTIC GUIDELINES BASED ON CONDITION

As mentioned earlier, the specific gastrointestinal condition and diagnosis along with the species-specific anatomy and physiology dictate the ideal treatment plan. Key therapeutic points are similar for rabbits, guinea pigs, and chinchillas for many of the conditions. Listed are the most common gastrointestinal conditions based on species.

Gastrointestinal Diseases of Rabbits

1. Ileus/hypomotility
2. Trichobezoars
3. Bacterial enteritis and diarrhea
4. Mucoid enteropathy
5. Parasitic enteritis
6. Gastric and intestinal ulcers
7. Dysbiosis and antibiotic-related enterotoxemia
8. Dental disease
9. Obstructive gastrointestinal disease
10. Hepatic lipidosis
11. Viral enteritis
12. Neoplasia
13. Liver lobe torsion

Gastrointestinal Diseases of Guinea Pigs

1. Gastric dilation and volvulus
2. Ileus
3. Bacterial enteritis
4. Parasitic enteritis
5. Fecal impaction
6. Hepatic lipidosis
7. Neoplasia
8. Obstructive disease
9. Dental disease

Gastrointestinal Diseases of Chinchillas

1. Diarrhea/soft stools
2. Bacterial enteritis
3. Dysbiosis and antibiotic-related enterotoxemia
4. Gas distention of stomach or intestinal system (tympany)
5. Constipation
6. Rectal prolapse
7. Intussusception
8. Megaesophagus
9. Dental disease
10. Parasitic enteritis

SUMMARY

The prognosis for the exotic mammal patient with gastrointestinal disease is dependent on the duration of the condition, patient age, stability at the time of presentation, and the specific diagnosis. In general, for gastrointestinal conditions, the timing of the diagnosis and initiation of treatment can be crucial in determining patient outcome. Many exotic mammal patients are presented to the veterinarian late in the disease process. This situation can make positive response to treatment or recovery challenging. Surgical conditions such as true gastrointestinal obstruction can have a good outcome if diagnosed early and if the patient is stable before surgery.

REFERENCES

1. Capello V, Lennox AM. Rabbit: abnormalities of the abdomen. In: Capello V, Lennox AM, editors. Clinical radiology of exotic companion mammals. Ames (IA): Wiley-Blackwell; 2008. p. 106–17.
2. DeCubellis J, Graham J. Gastrointestinal disease in guinea pigs and rabbits. Vet Clin North Am Exot Anim Pract 2013;16(2):421–35.
3. Harcourt-Brown F. The rabbit consultation. In: Harcourt-Brown F, editor. Textbook of rabbit medicine. Boston: Butterworth Heinemann; 2002. p. 52–93.
4. Longley LA. Rabbit anaesthesia. In: Longley LA, editor. Anaesthesia of exotic pets. London: Elsevier Saunders; 2008. p. 36–58.
5. Harcourt-Brown F. Anaesthesia and analgesia. In: Harcourt-Brown F, editor. Textbook of rabbit medicine. Boston: Butterworth Heinemann; 2002. p. 113–39.
6. Graham J, Mader DR. Basic approach to veterinary care. In: Quesenberry KE, Carpenter JW, editors. Ferrets, rabbits & rodents: clinical medicine & surgery. 3rd edition. St Louis (MO): Elsevier Saunders; 2012. p. 174–82.
7. Reusch B. Rabbit gastroenterology. Vet Clin North Am Exot Anim Pract 2005;8(2): 351–75.

8. Mans C, Donnelly TM. Disease problems of chinchillas. In: Quesenberry KE, Carpenter JW, editors. Ferrets, rabbits & rodents: clinical medicine & surgery. 3rd edition. St Louis (MO): Elsevier Saunders; 2012. p. 311–25.
9. Hawkins MG, Bishop CR. Disease problems of guinea pigs. In: Quesenberry KE, Carpenter JW, editors. Ferrets, rabbits & rodents: clinical medicine & surgery. 3rd edition. St Louis (MO): Elsevier Saunders; 2012. p. 295–310.
10. Oglesbee BL, Jenkins JR. Gastrointestinal diseases of rabbits. In: Quesenberry KE, Carpenter JW, editors. Ferrets, rabbits & rodents: clinical medicine & surgery. 3rd edition. St Louis (MO): Elsevier Saunders; 2012. p. 192–204.
11. Oglesbee BL. Gastrointestinal hypomotility and gastrointestinal stasis in rabbits. In: Oglesbee BL, editor. Blackwells's five-minute veterinary consult: small mammal. 2nd edition. West Sussex (United Kingdom): Wiley-Blackwell; 2011. p. 425–8.
12. Vella D. Intestinal disorders in rabbits. In: Mayer J, Donnelly TM, editors. Clinical veterinary advisor birds and exotic pets. St Louis (MO): Elsevier Saunders; 2013. p. 385–90.
13. Krempels D, Cotter M, Stanzione G. Ileus in domestic rabbits. Exotic DVM 2000; 2.4:19–21.
14. Fisher PG. Exotic mammal gastrointestinal disease. In: Proceedings Western Veterinary Conference. Las Vegas (NV): Western Veterinary Conference; 2011. p. 1–11.
15. Johnson DH. The gastrointestinal tract of the rabbit: health and disease (Part 1). Proceedings American Board Veterinary Practitioners. San Antonio (TX): American Board of Veterinary Practitioners; 2012. p. 1–8.
16. Johnson DH. The gastrointestinal tract of the rabbit: health and disease (part 2). Proceedings American Board Veterinary Practitioners. San Antonio (TX): American Board of Veterinary Practitioners; 2012. p. 9–18.
17. Girling SJ. Fundamentals of rabbit GI husbandry and disease. Proceedings London Vet Show. London: Proceedings of London Vet Show; 2011.
18. Hoefer HL. Gastrointestinal diseases of rabbits. Proceedings Atlantic Coast Veterinary Conference. Atlantic City (NJ): Atlantic Coast Veterinary Conference; 2010. p. 1–4.
19. Ritzman TK. Use of a vascular access port (VAP) in a chinchilla (*Chinchilla lanigera*) for chemotherapy. Proceedings Assoc Exotic Animal Veterinarians Conference. Indianapolis (IN): Association of Exotic Mammal Veterinarians; 2013.
20. Barter LS. Rabbit analgesia. Vet Clin North Am Exot Anim Pract 2011;14(1): 93–104.
21. Plumb DC. Plumb's veterinary drug handbook. 7th edition. Ames (IA): Wiley-Blackwell; 2011.
22. Carpenter JW, Marion CJ, editors. Exotic animal formulary. 4th edition. St Louis (MO): Elsevier Saunders; 2013.
23. Carpenter JW, Pollock CG, Koch DE, et al. Single and multiple-dose pharmacokinetics of meloxicam after oral administration to the rabbit (*Oryctolagus cuniculus*). J Zoo Wildl Med 2009;40(4):601–6.
24. Cooper CS, Metcalf-Pate KA, Barat CE, et al. Comparison of side effects between buprenorphine and meloxicam used postoperatively in Dutch belted rabbits (*Oryctolagus cuniculus*). J Am Assoc Lab Anim Sci 2009;48(3):279–85.
25. Souza MJ, Greenacre CB, Cox SK. Pharmacokinetics of orally administered tramadol in domestic rabbits (*Oryctolagus cuniculus*). Am J Vet Res 2008;69(8): 979–82.
26. Remillard RL. Parenteral nutrition support in rabbits and ferrets. Journal of Exotic Pet Medicine 2006;15(4):248–54.

Liver Lobe Torsion in Pet Rabbits
Clinical Consequences, Diagnosis, and Treatment

Jennifer Graham, DVM, DABVP (Avian/Exotic Companion Mammal), DACZM[a,b,*],
Jessica Basseches, DVM, DACVR[c]

KEYWORDS

- Gastrointestinal disease • Rabbit • Stasis • Liver torsion

KEY POINTS

- Liver lobe torsion is a relatively uncommon presentation in pet rabbits.
- Rabbits with liver lobe torsion generally present with nonspecific signs of gastrointestinal stasis.
- Delay in diagnosis and surgical correction of liver lobe torsion in rabbits may be associated with death.
- Ultrasound examination is generally diagnostic for liver lobe torsion in rabbits.
- Rabbits may survive liver lobe torsion with medical management only.
- One of the authors has documented 16 cases of liver torsion in rabbits at a single referral institution in 5 years.

INTRODUCTION

Liver lobe torsion is rarely reported in any species, but reports exist in people, horses, dogs, pigs, otters, rats, mice, and rabbits.[1–26] In veterinary medicine, liver lobe torsion is most commonly described in dogs.[4,13,14,16,19] Acute venous infarction and lobar hepatic necrosis occur and can result in effusion, hemoabdomen, shock, and death. Disseminated intravascular coagulation has been reported as a result of bacterial toxin and ischemic by-product release.

Although the cause of liver lobe torsion is unknown, predisposing factors are thought to include surgical or external trauma, congenital absence of hepatic ligaments, or dilation of abdominal organs.[10,16,19,26] It is also possible that liver lobe

The authors have nothing to disclose.
[a] Department of Zoological Companion Animal Medicine, Cummings School of Veterinary Medicine at Tufts University, 200 Westboro Road, North Grafton, MA 01536, USA; [b] Department of Comparative Medicine, University of Washington School of Medicine, 1959 Northeast Pacific Street, Seattle, WA 98195, USA; [c] Center for Animal Referral and Emergency Services, 2010 Cabot Boulevard, Langhorne, PA 19047, USA
* Corresponding author. Department of Zoological Companion Animal Medicine, Cummings School of Veterinary Medicine at Tufts University, 200 Westboro Road, North Grafton, MA 01536.
E-mail address: Jennifer.Graham@Tufts.edu

pathology including parasitic and bacterial infection or neoplasia could contribute to an increased incidence of torsion.[4,16,27] The left lateral lobe is reportedly most prone to torsion in species other than rabbits and thought to be related to its relatively larger size, increased mobility, and separation from other lobes.[8,15] In rabbits, the caudate liver lobe is reportedly prone to displacement, theoretically because of its narrow attachment to the dorsal hilar region of the liver.[27] A recent retrospective review of 16 cases of liver lobe torsion in rabbits showed that the caudate lobe was torsed in 63% of cases.[1] In addition, a literature review of 29 cases (including the 16 from the retrospective review) described 18 of 29 rabbits (62%) with torsion of the caudate lobe.

The most common signs in dogs with liver lobe torsion are nonspecific signs including lethargy, anorexia, vomiting, collapse, or sudden death. Increases in hepatic enzyme activities are typical in cases of liver lobe torsion in dogs.[8] Although radiographs are generally not diagnostic for live lobe torsion in most species, ultrasound with Doppler assessment of hepatic vessels may be useful to diagnose liver lobe torsion in dogs, although reports differ on this point.[8,28] Prompt diagnosis and liver lobectomy are vital for cases of liver lobe torsion.

CLINICAL CONSEQUENCES

Liver lobe torsion has been reported as an incidental finding in rabbits. Three cases of liver lobe torsion were reported during necropsy of 984 laboratory rabbits that died of pasteurellosis with no reported abdominal signs.[23] Two of the rabbits in the report had atrophied lobes, while the third rabbit appeared to have a recent torsion. This report suggested that liver lobe torsion is likely to occur infrequently in rabbits and that rabbits may survive after torsion of a lobe. A recent retrospective of 16 cases of liver lobe torsion in rabbits revealed that 3 of 7 (43%) rabbits survived torsion with supportive care measures alone.[1] The authors documented a rabbit over a several year period with an incidental finding of an atrophied liver lobe on ultrasound possibly secondary to a previous torsion.

Liver lobe torsion has also been suspected as a cause of death in rabbits. A report of a rabbit found dead in its cage identified liver lobe torsion as the presumptive cause of death.[25] Four out of 7 rabbits (57%) treated with supportive care measures only died as a result of complications due to liver lobe torsion in the retrospective study by Graham and colleagues.[1] Based on this information, as well as outcomes reported in other species, it was concluded that untreated cases of liver lobe torsion may result in death of the rabbit.

SIGNALMENT

Based on the retrospective study by Graham and colleagues,[1] the median age of presentation for rabbits with liver torsion was 5.15 years. There was no sex predilection. The median body weight was 2.57 kg. Eleven of the rabbits were Mini Lops, and other breeds included: 1 Dutch, 1 Holland Lop, 1 American Fuzzy Lop, and 2 mixed breeds. Most Lops in the report were noted to be white with brown spots (**Fig. 1**). Although an attempt was made to identify sources of rabbits, most had been rescued, so it was impossible to try and determine a common breeder. Determination of lineage could be helpful to prove a genetic predisposition. As an aside, cases of hepatic torsion reports in rabbits on file with 2 specialty pathology services were evaluated to determine if there appeared to be a breed predisposition, and there was not.

Many of the rabbits with liver torsion in the retrospective study by Graham and colleagues had a history of prior gastrointestinal (GI) stasis, and one of these rabbits had

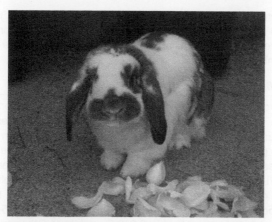

Fig. 1. Image of a Mini Lop rabbit that was diagnosed with liver lobe torsion. Most Lops with liver lobe torsions identified by the authors have been white with brown spots.

a prior gastrotomy. There is a suspected relationship between gastric dilatation-volvulus and liver lobe torsion in dogs, and prophylactic gastropexy is recommended at the time of liver lobectomy in dogs.[8] Supporting hepatic ligaments in rabbits are similar to those found in dogs, so it is possible that stretching of the left triangular ligament in association with gastric dilation could potentially predispose to liver lobe torsion.

HISTORY AND PHYSICAL EXAMINATION

The most common complaints on presentation of rabbits with liver lobe torsion in the report by Graham and colleagues[1] included anorexia (94%), lethargy (56%), decreased fecal production (38%), inappropriate urination and defecation (25%), crouched or hunched body position (25%), hiding behavior (13%), and soft stools (13%). These findings are typical for what is generally seen in GI stasis and most cases were initially suspected to be primary GI stasis. The median duration of clinical signs prior to presentation was 1 day.

The most common physical examination findings in rabbits with liver lobe torsion in the report by Graham and colleagues[1] included abdominal pain (75%), dehydration (38%), increased intestinal gas (31%), tachypnea (25%), decreased borborygmi (19%), dull mentation (19%), hypothermia (19%), and a mass effect or palpable liver edge in the cranial abdomen (19%). Other physical examination findings included tachycardia (13%) and an elevated body temperature (6%). Clinicians experienced with rabbit abdominal palpation may be more likely to take note of the mass effect or palpable liver edge in the cranial abdomen based on comparison of physical examination findings noted by receiving emergency doctors when compared to notes taken on the patient after transfer to DABVP-ECM practitioners.

DIAGNOSIS
Complete Blood Count

A complete blood count (CBC) was performed in 14 of 16 rabbits in the report by Graham and colleagues.[1] The most common hematologic abnormality was anemia (68%). The median packed cell volume was 28.2%. Most rabbits sampled had evidence of red blood cell fragmentation including acanthocytosis, schistocytosis, and echinocytosis. Nucleated red blood cells were recorded in 3 rabbits, and increased polychromasia was noted in 2 rabbits. Thrombocytopenia (n = 7) and leukopenia (n = 2) were also noted. Interestingly, 2 rabbits had subjectively prolonged clotting times following venipuncture; one of these rabbits died, and one was euthanized because of declining condition.

Biochemistry Profile

A biochemistry profile was performed in 15 of 16 rabbits in the report by Graham and colleagues.[1] The most common serum biochemical abnormalities were elevated levels of alanine aminotransferase (n = 14), alkaline phosphatase (n = 11), aspartate aminotransferase (n = 7), blood urea nitrogen (n = 8), and creatinine (n = 4). The median level of these analytes relative to reference ranges were: alanine aminotransferase, 615.5 IU/L (reference range, 14–80 IU/L); alkaline phosphatase, 140 IU/L (reference range, 4–16 IU/L); aspartate aminotransferase, 931 IU/L (reference range, 14–113 IU/L); blood urea nitrogen, 32 mg/dL (reference range 15–30 mg/dL); and creatinine, 1.4 mg/dL (reference range, 0.8–2.5 mg/dL).[29] Other serum biochemical abnormalities included elevated levels of glucose (n = 3), cholesterol (n = 2), bilirubin (n = 1), globulin (n = 1), and phosphorous (n = 1), and decreased levels of total protein (n = 3), potassium (n = 2), bicarbonate (n = 2), globulin (n = 1), and phosphorous (n = 1).

Radiographs

Abdominal radiographs were obtained in 12 of 16 rabbits in the report by Graham and colleagues.[1] Rounded liver margins or hepatomegaly were noted in 3 cases, and increased gastric or intestinal gas, suggestive of gastrointestinal stasis or obstruction, was noted in 11 cases (**Fig. 2**). Loss of serosal detail, free peritoneal fluid, or an obscured liver border was demonstrated in 3 cases.

Ultrasound

Abdominal ultrasonography was performed in 14 rabbits (88%) in the report by Graham and colleagues[1] and was diagnostic for liver lobe torsion in all cases. Common ultrasonographic findings included hepatomegaly or an abnormally large liver lobe, rounded lobar margins, mixed liver parenchymal echogenicity, hyperechoic perihepatic mesentery, and free peritoneal fluid. Color flow Doppler revealed a lack of or decreased blood flow in the affected liver lobe(s) in all cases (**Fig. 3**).

TREATMENT
Surgery

Exploratory celiotomy and liver lobectomy were performed in 9 rabbits in the report by Graham and colleagues.[1] Surgical correction (**Fig. 4**) involved circumferential ligature occlusion of the lobe and transection distal to the ligatures. Ligation was performed with a Surgitie instrument (Surgitie Loop With Polysorb Suture - EI-20-L individual suture, Covidien, Mansfield, Massachusetts) (n = 5), sutures (n = 3), or metal clips (n = 1). In 4 of the 9 rabbits, liver biopsies were submitted for aerobic and anaerobic bacterial cultures, and 1 biopsy yielded growth of *Staphylococcus epidermidis*. Histologic examination of the affected liver lobes was performed in 9 cases and was consistent with acute or chronic liver lobe torsion in all cases. The torsed liver lobe was recorded in the medical record of all cases at the time of ultrasound, surgery, or postmortem examination; affected lobes included the caudate lobe (63%), right lateral lobe (31%), left lateral lobe (13%), and right medial lobe (6%). Two cases had more than 1 affected liver lobe; one had torsed caudate and right lateral lobes, and another had torsed left lateral and right lateral lobes. No intraoperative complications were noted.

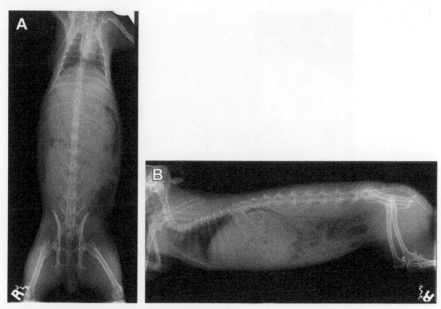

Fig. 2. (*A, B*) Lateral and ventrodorsal radiographic projections of a rabbit with a caudate and right liver lobe torsion. Note the gastric distention with ingesta and increased volume of gas and intestinal content, suggestive of gastric stasis and paralytic Ileus.

All rabbits treated surgically survived. Postoperative complications occurred in 2 of the rabbits undergoing hepatectomy and included elevated body temperature (n = 2) and loose stools (n = 1) that resolved uneventfully. The median duration of hospital stay for postsurgical rabbits was 4 days (range, 3–6 days).

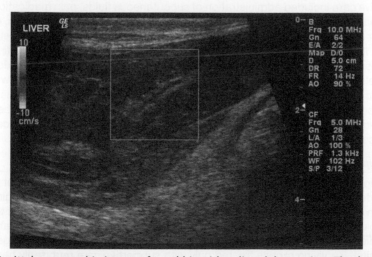

Fig. 3. Sagittal sonographic image of a rabbit with a liver lobe torsion. The box over a portion of the torsed lobe represents the region of sampling and demonstrates a lack of blood flow to the affected liver lobe. Note the decreased echogenicity of the lobe and the surrounding hyperechoic fat, common findings seen on ultrasound of liver lobe torsions in rabbits.

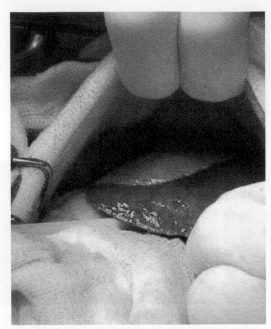

Fig. 4. Intraoperative photograph of a rabbit with a liver lobe torsion. Note the mottled and dark appearance of the ischemic, torsed liver lobe that is dorsal to a normal liver lobe.

Supportive Care

Seven of the 16 rabbits were treated with supportive care measures only in the report by Graham and colleagues.[1] Of these, 3 rabbits (43%) survived. The median hospital stay for rabbits treated with only with supportive care was 2 days (range, 1–3 days). Supportive care included administration of subcutaneous fluids, pain medications, antimicrobials, supplemental feeding, and prokinetic agents. In 4 of these cases, owners opted for supportive care after declining surgical treatment. Diagnosis was delayed in 2 cases. In the first instance (and the first torsion case on record during the timeline), diagnosis was not made until postmortem examination. The rabbit had toxic blood lead levels and decompensated despite chelation therapy, and a necropsy was performed to search for underlying disease. In the second instance, the rabbit was initially treated on an emergency basis, and no diagnostics were performed until the rabbit presented again 2 days later. Liver lobe torsion was then diagnosed and surgical treatment recommended, but the rabbit died prior to surgery.

Follow-up

Follow-up examinations and re-evaluation of CBC and/or serum biochemical profiles were performed on 3 of the surviving rabbits 1 week to 2 months after the original presentation in the report by Graham and colleagues.[1] In all instances, results of the clinicopathologic tests were normal or improved relative to results of the same tests at the time of diagnosis. Follow-up information was obtained for all rabbits discharged from the hospital. Surviving rabbits treated only with supportive care reportedly had multiple episodes of recurrent GI stasis within the first 1 to 2 months following hospitalization. One of these rabbits has had ongoing reports of GI stasis that have been responsive to medical management. All rabbits that survived to the time of discharge (n = 12) are reportedly stable and have had no recurrent episodes of liver lobe torsion.

ACKNOWLEDGMENTS

The authors would like to acknowledge Angell Animal Medical Center for provision of medical records for the rabbits in this report.

REFERENCES

1. Graham JE, Orcutt CJ, Casale SA, et al. Liver lobe torsion in rabbits: 16 cases (2007–2012). Journal of Exotic Pet Medicine. in press.
2. Bentz KJ, Burgess BA, Lohmann KL, et al. Hepatic lobe torsion in a horse. Can Vet J 2009;50:283–6.
3. Bhandal J, Kuzma A, Starrak G. Spontaneous left medial liver lobe torsion and left lateral lobe infarction in a Rottweiler. Can Vet J 2008;49:1002–4.
4. Downs MO, Miller MA, Cross AR, et al. Liver lobe torsion and liver abscess in a dog. J Am Vet Med Assoc 1998;212:678–80.
5. Evering W, Edwards JF. Hepatic lobe deformity in a rabbit. Lab Anim 1992;21:14–6.
6. Fitzgerald AL, Fitzgerald SD. Hepatic lobe torsion in a New Zealand White rabbit. Canine Pract 1992;17:16–9.
7. Hamir AN. Torsion of the liver in a sow. Vet Rec 1980;106:362–3.
8. Hinkle Schwartz SG, Mitchell SL, Keating JH, et al. Liver lobe torsion in dogs: 13 cases (1995–2004). J Am Vet Med Assoc 2006;228:242–7.
9. Lee K, Yamada K, Hirokawa H, et al. Liver lobe torsion in a Shih-tzu dog. J Small Anim Pract 2009;50:157.
10. McConkey S, Briggs C, Solano M, et al. Liver torsion and associated bacterial peritonitis in a dog. Can Vet J 1997;38:438–9.
11. Morin M, Sauvageau R, Phaneuf JB, et al. Torsion of abdominal organs in sows: a report of 36 cases. Can Vet J 1984;25:440–2.
12. Saunders R, Redrobe S, Barr F, et al. Liver lobe torsion in rabbits. J Small Anim Pract 2009;50:562.
13. Scheck MG. Liver lobe torsion in a dog. Can Vet J 2007;48:423–5.
14. Sonnenfield JM, Armbrust LJ, Radlinsky MA, et al. Radiographic and ultrasonographic findings of liver lobe torsion in a dog. Vet Radiol Ultrasound 2001;42:344–6.
15. Stanke NJ, Graham JE, Orcutt CJ, et al. Successful outcome of hepatectomy for liver lobe torsion in four domestic rabbits. J Am Vet Med Assoc 2011;238:1176–83.
16. Swann HM, Brown DC. Hepatic lobe torsion in 3 dogs and a cat. Vet Surg 2001;30:482–6.
17. Taylor HR, Staff CD. Clinical techniques: successful management of liver lobe torsion in a domestic rabbit (Oryctolagus cuniculus) by surgical lobectomy. Journal of Exotic Pet Medicine 2007;16:175–8.
18. Tennett-Brown B, Mudge MC, Hardy J, et al. Liver lobe torsion in six horses. J Am Vet Med Assoc 2012;241:615–20.
19. Tomlinson J, Black A. Liver lobe torsion in a dog. J Am Vet Med Assoc 1983;183:225–6.
20. Turner TA, Brown CA, Wilson JH, et al. Hepatic lobe torsion as a cause of colic in a horse. Vet Surg 1993;22:301–4.
21. von Pfeil DJ, Jutkowitz LA, Hauptman J, et al. Left lateral and left middle liver lobe torsion in a Saint Bernard puppy. J Am Anim Hosp Assoc 2006;42:381–5.
22. Warns-Petit ES. Liver lobe torsion in an oriental small-clawed otter (Aonyx cinerea). Vet Rec 2001;148:212–3.

23. Weisbroth SH. Torsion of the caudate lobe of the liver in the domestic rabbit (Oryctolagus). Vet Pathol 1975;12:13–5.
24. Wenger S, Barrett EL, Pearson GR, et al. Liver lobe torsion in three adult rabbits. J Small Anim Pract 2009;50:301–5.
25. Wilson RB, Holscher MA, Sly DL. Liver lobe torsion in a rabbit. Lab Anim Sci 1987; 37:506–7.
26. Woolfe DT, English B. Torsion of the left lateral and papillary lobes of the liver in a pup—a case report. J Am Vet Med Assoc 1959;134:458.
27. Vella D, Donnelly TM. Basic anatomy, physiology, and husbandry. In: Quesenberry KE, Carpenter JW, editors. Ferrets, rabbits, and rodents: clinical medicine and surgery. 3rd edition. Philadelphia: WB Saunders; 2012. p. 157–73.
28. Singh M, Foster A, Marchevsky A, et al. Hepatic lobe torsion and gastric-dilatation volvulus in a dog. Aust Vet Pract 2002;32:174–8.
29. Fiorello C, Divers S. Rabbits. In: Carpenter J, Marion C, editors. Exotic animal formulary. 4th edition. St Louis (MO): Saunders; 2013. p. 517–57.

Update on the Diagnosis and Management of *Macrorhabdus Ornithogaster* (Formerly Megabacteria) in Avian Patients

David N. Phalen, DVM, PhD, Dipl. ABVP (Avian)

KEYWORDS

* Bird * Diagnosis * *Macrorhabdus ornithogaster* * Treatment

KEY POINTS

* *Macrorhabdus ornithogaster* is a yeast found only at the junction between the ventriculus and proventriculus in birds.
* *M ornithogaster* can infect a wide range of birds.
* Infection with *M ornithogaster* is often subclinical but can also result in gastrointestinal signs.
* Direct observation of the organism in the feces is a specific but somewhat insensitive means of diagnosis.
* At least three antifungal drugs are reported to be effective for treatment of *M ornithogaster* but resistance to one or more of these drugs may occur.

INTRODUCTION

Macrorhabdus ornithogaster is an anamorphic Ascomycetes yeast that grows only at the junction of the proventriculus and ventriculus in birds.[1] It can infect many species of birds.[2–4] There is convincing evidence *M ornithogaster* can cause disease in its host but it is also clear that many birds live with this organism without obvious signs. The only effective treatments for *M ornithogaster* are a few antifungal drugs and these drugs do not always lend themselves to large-scale flock treatment. Because *M ornithogaster* was thought to be a bacterium (Megabacteria) for more than 20 years[4,5] many assumptions about this organism's biology have subsequently proven to be untrue.[1] Continued referencing of some of these flawed studies and anecdotal reports often creates confusion for veterinarians and bird owners alike.

Faculty of Veterinary Science, University of Sydney, 425 Werombi Road, Camden, New South Wales 2570, Australia
E-mail address: david.phalen@sydney.edu.au

Vet Clin Exot Anim 17 (2014) 203–210
http://dx.doi.org/10.1016/j.cvex.2014.01.005
1094-9194/14/$ – see front matter © 2014 Elsevier Inc. All rights reserved.

HOST RANGE

The reported host range of *M ornithogaster* includes a wide range of psittacine birds, passerine birds, poultry, and other species. It has a worldwide distribution and it is found in both wild and captive birds.[2,3,6–17]

The species of psittacine birds most commonly infected with *M ornithogaster* are the budgerigar (*Melopsittacus undulatus*), lovebirds (*Agapornis* sp), and to lesser extent cockatiels (*Nymphicus hollandicus*).[3–6,8,9,11,16–19] Infection has also been reported as common in parrotlets (*Forpus* sp).[17] In wild Australian birds, the organism is commonly found in recently fledged Galahs (*Eolophus roseicapilla*) and Corellas (*Cacatua* sp) with chronic diarrheal disease and weight loss. These birds have other intestinal parasites and at least some have concurrent infections with the Psittacine Beak and Feather Disease Virus.[20] The full host range of *M ornithogaster* in Psittacine birds is unknown and infection should be considered in any species of Psittacine bird presenting with gastrointestinal signs.

Passerines infected with *M ornithogaster* include pet canaries (*Serinus canaria*), zebra finches (*Taeniopygia guttata*), and Gouldian finches (*Erythrura gouldiae*).[2–4,8,20] It has also been found in a range of wild European finches and the sisken (*Carduelis spinus*),[10,11] as well as in feral European goldfinches (*Carduelis carduelis*) and wild-caught feral European goldfinches and green finches (*Carduelis chloris*) captured for the pet trade in Australia.[20]

M ornithogaster infections have now been reported in chickens (*Gallus gallus*) on four continents: Europe, North and South America, and Australia.[17,21–23] Other gallinaceous birds reported to be infected with *M ornithogaster* include the gray partridge (*Perdix perdix*),[14] the Japanese quail (*Coturnix japonica*),[12,13] domestic turkey (*Meleagris gallopavo*),[11,13] chukar partridge (*Alectoris chukar*), and guinea fowl (genus and species not reported).[13] Infection has also been reported in ducks, geese, and ibis although no supporting evidence on how the diagnosis was made in ibis was provided. Recently, *M ornithogaster* has been reported in captive-raised greater rheas (*Rhea americana*).[13] Morphologically, these organisms are consistent with those that have been reported in other species. However, they remain to be characterized by molecular techniques.

There are two reports of an organism resembling *M ornithogaster* infecting the upper respiratory tract of a dog and a cat.[24,25] These organisms were never described and given that *M ornithogaster* is microaerophilic, their growth on a respiratory epithelium does not seem plausible. Recent infection attempts in mice provide additional evidence that *M ornithogaster* cannot grow in mammals.[26]

Isolation attempts from stomach contents of greater rheas using growth conditions that are inconsistent with the metabolic requirements of *M ornithogaster* have resulted in the isolation of a small motile organism, which the investigators suggest is *M ornithogaster*. This uncharacterized organism has been shown to be able to colonize the stomach of mice.[13] Given that this organism grows in conditions that are incompatible for *M ornithogaster* growth, that it has morphologic characteristics that have never been seen in *M ornithogaster* either in vivo or in vitro, and that it has never been characterized genetically, it is the author's opinion that the conclusion that this organism is *M ornithogaster* is premature and is probably incorrect.

DIAGNOSIS
Clinical Signs

The clinical signs of *M ornithogaster* in birds have been well described.[2,6–8,12,17–19,27,28] Vomiting, diarrhea, and chronic weight loss are the most common signs described across a range of species. Disease has been seen in young birds and adult birds. The disease in budgerigars occurs most commonly in middle-aged birds.[27,28] An acute hemorrhagic disease has been reported in parrotlets.[17] Weight loss, anorexia, melena, and anemia are commonly seen in cockatiels and occasionally in other species that have gastric ulceration secondary to *M ornithogaster* infection. Canaries and other finches with *M ornithogaster* are often found dead but are generally emaciated, suggesting that they had been ill for at least a few days before death.[2,4,10]

Diagnosis in the Live Bird

Detection of *M ornithogaster* infection in the live bird is most commonly done by microscopic examination of the feces. Feces made into a slurry with water or saline can be scanned for *M ornithogaster* using 40× magnification. Alternately, fecal smears can be stained with a quick stain or Gram stain. A rapid way of concentrating *M ornithogaster* and separating it from other solid mater in the feces is to homogenize a dropping with approximately 20 times its volume of physiologic saline in a small tube, let it sit for 10 seconds, and then examine a small drop of the suspension collected from the meniscus. Because *M ornithogaster* takes longer to settle than most other material in the feces they are more easily seen in wet preparations after this treatment. A polymerase chain reaction (PCR) assay to detect *M ornithogaster* in the feces is also available in North America (Veterinary Molecular Diagnostics, Milford, Ohio, USA).

M ornithogaster are long, slender, straight stiff rods with rounded ends when they are found in the feces (**Fig. 1**). In some circumstances, the long rods may bend slightly in a gentle curve. Y-shaped organisms may be seen but these are extremely rare. Viewed directly in a wet mount, small oblong refractile structures found at regular intervals are readily seen. These structures are nuclei. The nuclei stain with Giemsa stains (**Fig. 2**). *M ornithogaster* range in length from 20 to 80 μm and are consistently

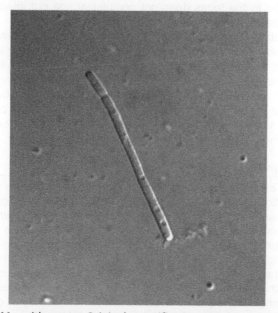

Fig. 1. Unstained *M ornithogaster.* Original magnification 100×.

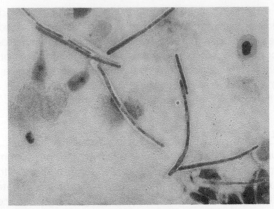

Fig. 2. *M ornithogaster* stained with Gram stain. Original magnification 100×. (*From* Phalen DN. Diagnosis and management of *Macrorhabdus ornithogaster* (formerly megabacteria). Vet Clin Exot Anim 2005;8:302; with permission.)

2 to 3 μm across. They often stain poorly with quick stains and the Gram stain and, instead of staining uniformly, will only pick up small droplets of the stain. When they do stain well, they are gram-positive and stain dark blue with quick stains (see **Fig. 1**). Unlike bacteria and other yeasts, the contents of the cell stain, but not the cell wall. It is the author's impression that they do not stick well to glass slides unless the slide has been heat fixed. It is also the author's impression that heat fixing makes them more likely to stain uniformly.

Birds infected with *M ornithogaster* may shed the organism in low numbers, in large numbers, or not at all.[15,17] It has been the author's experience that most birds that are exhibiting disease as the result of *M ornithogaster* infection will be shedding large numbers of organisms. However, this may not always be the case and the absence of *M ornithogaster* in the feces does not completely rule out infection or infection and associated disease.

There can be other things in the feces that resemble *M ornithogaster*. An unknown structure commonly seen by the author in the droppings of many birds is approximately the size of *M ornithogaster* but has a straight, not rounded, terminal end that appears to be the result of the structure breaking off of something larger. *M ornithogaster* always has rounded ends. Filamentous gram-positive bacteria can also approach the size of *M ornithogaster*. These bacteria, however, are often segmented, are thinner than *M ornithogaster*, and generally curve back and forth and thus are readily distinguished from *M ornithogaster*.

Postmortem Diagnosis

M ornithogaster infection is readily made at postmortem. A saline preparation of a scraping of junction (isthmus) of the proventriculus and the ventriculus will demonstrate the organisms and they will generally be abundant. *M ornithogaster* is also readily demonstrated in hematoxylin and eosin stained sections of the isthmus. They are eosinophilic and are found forming the characteristic log-jam patterns on the surface of and between the mucosal glands.[3,4] They stain with silver stains and the periodic acid shift stain.[1] Showing that the *M ornithogaster* infection contributed to the cause of the bird's death, however, requires more proof than just finding the organism. Budgerigars and passerines with disease caused by *M ornithogaster* will grossly have a thickened mucosa of the proventriculus and there will be increased mucous in the lumen.[2,3,10,18,27,29] Some birds may have one or more bleeding ulcers of the proventriculus. In birds with clinical signs caused by *M ornithogaster* infection, growth extends beyond the isthmus into the proventriculus and the koilin of ventriculus and may disrupt the structure of the koilin. A lymphoplasmacytic inflammation is common in birds with heavy *M ornithogaster* growth but is less likely in birds with minimal superficial colonization of the organism.[30]

Growth In Vitro

M ornithogaster is readily grown in vitro given the correct substrate and conditions. It must be provided with a microaerophilic environment and grown in a medium with a pH between 3 and 4. Traditional cell culture media containing up to 20% fetal bovine serum and 1% to 5% glucose or sucrose has been shown to support its growth. Its optimal growth temperature is 42°C. Addition of antibiotics to the growth media is recommended to prevent the overgrowth of bacteria. It can be cultured from isthmus scrapings or from feces.[31]

TREATMENT

There are few treatment trials done in birds with *M ornithogaster* infection.[17,20,29,32–36] In many of these trials, the measure of successful treatment was the cessation of *M ornithogaster* shedding in the feces,[33,34] as opposed to the less common trial in which treated birds were killed and the stomach examined directly.[29,32,35,36] Although it is likely that the cessation of shedding may be the result of a cure, it is also possible that some of these treated birds remained infected at low levels.

Amphotericin B

Amphotericin B is used widely to treat *M ornithogaster* and seems to be effective and safe when administered orally by gavage and, in some circumstances, in the water. Various dosages have been recommended.[33] The author has used 100 mg/kg, twice a day for 14 days with direct oral administration, but has been gradually reducing the amount and is now using 25 mg/kg, twice a day for 14 days with apparent success. Success of treatment has been judged by the rapid cessation of *M ornithogaster* shedding and resolution of signs. Amphotericin B can be purchased as a powder and compounded into a formula that can be given orally or it can be obtained as a 2.5% water soluble powder. The water soluble product used in drinking water at 0.9 mg/mL stopped shedding in infected budgerigars in a small scale trial of 10 birds.[34] The author has had inconsistent results with this product in sick birds of various species, possibly because they do not consume enough water to achieve an effective dosage rate or for other unknown reasons.[17] It is the author's preference to mix this product with lactulose and administer it directly into the mouth of the sick bird using the previously described protocol. There is one report of resistance *M ornithogaster* to amphotericin B.[33] How widespread resistance may be is not known.

Nystatin

The ability of nystatin to kill *M ornithogaster* may vary from strain to strain. In vitro trials by Bradley and colleagues[35] showed that *M ornithogaster* was sensitive to nystatin at concentrations of 0.1 U/ml (Chan P, personal communication, 2012).[37] In one clinical trial, the investigators also saw a cessation of *M ornithogaster* shedding after treatment with nystatin.[33] In a recent study, a flock of budgerigars was treated with nystatin at 3,500,000 IU per liter of drinking water for 2 days, then 2,000,000 IU per liter for 28 days.[29] Some birds in this study were euthanized after the end of treatment and were found free of infection. Resistance to nystatin by some strains of *M ornithogaster* is likely based on clinical trials done by other investigators, so birds treated with nystatin should be monitored closely to see if shedding ceases.[33]

Low Toxic Antifungal Chemicals

Research done by Bradley and colleagues[35] showed that *M ornithogaster* in vitro are highly sensitive to sodium and potassium benzoate and sodium sorbate. Treatment attempts with sodium benzoate in drinking water in live birds have been trialled by the author and others.[35] The author's experiences have not been uniformly successful and, in many cases, shedding and clinical signs have not resolved (Chan P, personal communication, 2012). The cause of the failure of treatment is not known; however, adequate consumption of the treated water may be to blame. In another trial in which a flock of breeding budgerigars were treated, *M ornithogaster* shedding stopped but deaths of some of the treated birds also occurred. The cause of the deaths was not determined but could have been the result of sodium toxicity. Water consumption in the treated budgerigars was very high because they were feeding young, it was the middle of the summer, and daytime temperatures were very high.[35] The use of potassium benzoate has not been trialled but it may be safer than sodium benzoate because it is more difficult to get potassium toxicity from ingested potassium than it is to get sodium toxicity from ingested sodium. The use of any of these chemicals requires additional research before they can be recommended for routine use. There are many potential sources of sodium and potassium benzoate. The product used by the author is purchased as a 99% pure product.

Other Antifungals

Fluconazole has been used to effectively treat to *M ornithogaster* in experimentally infected chickens at dosage of 100 mg/kg.[36] In trials in budgerigars, this dosage rate was found to be toxic and a lower dosage rate was not effective.[32] Gentian violet was found to prevent *M ornithogaster* growth in vitro.[37] However, gentian violet at moderate concentrations was found to be toxic to budgerigars (Phalen, unpublished information, 2005).

SUMMARY

M ornithogaster is found in a many species of birds around the world. It can be a significant cause of both morbidity and mortality. Detecting the infection in the live bird requires the direct observation of the organism in the feces or its detection by PCR; however, these assays are not sufficiently sensitive that a negative result rules out infection. Diagnosis is readily made at postmortem by examination of scrapings of the isthmus and histopathology of the proventriculus and ventriculus. The only consistently proven treatment of infected birds is direct oral administration of amphotericin B, although, nystatin and sodium benzoate may also be effective in some circumstances.

REFERENCES

1. Tomaszewski EK, Logan KE, Kurtzman CP, et al. Phylogenetic analysis indicates the 'megabacterium' of birds is a novel anamorphic ascomycetous yeast, *Macrorhabdus ornithogaster*, gen. nov., sp. nov. Int J Syst Evol Microbiol 2003;3:1201–5.
2. Dorrestein GM, Zwart P, Buitellaar MN. Problems arising from disease during the periods of breeding and rearing canaries and other aviary birds. Tijdschr Diergeneeskd 1980;105:535–43.

3. Hargreaves RC. A fungus commonly found in the proventriculus of small pet birds. In: 30th Western Poultry Disease Conference and 15th Poultry Health Symposium. University of California at Davis. Davis (CA). March 9–13, 1981. p. 75–6.
4. van Herck H, Duijser T, Zwart P, et al. A bacterial proventriculitis of canaries. Avian Pathol 1984;13:561–72.
5. Scanlan CM, Graham DL. Characterization of a gram-positive bacterium from the proventriculus of budgerigars (*Melopsittacus undulatus*). Avian Dis 1990;34:779–86.
6. Henderson GM, Gulland MD, Hawkey CM. Haematological findings in budgerigars with megabacterium and *Trichomonas* infections associated with 'going light'. Vet Rec 1988;123:492–4.
7. Huchzermeyer FW, Henton MM, Keffen RH. High mortality associated with megabacteriosis of proventriculus and gizzard in ostrich chicks. Vet Rec 1993;133:143–4.
8. Filippich LJ, O'Boyle DA, Webb R, et al. Megabacteria in birds in Australia. Aust Vet Prac 1993;23:72–6.
9. Ravelhofer K, Rotheneder R, Gareis M, et al. Megabacteriosis in different bird species. DVG Tag Vogelkr 1998;9:95–104.
10. Pennycott TW, Ross HM, MCLaren IM, et al. Causes of death of wild birds of the family *Fringillidae* in Britain. Vet Rec 1998;143:155–8.
11. Gerlach H. Megabacteriosis. Sem Avian Exotic Pet Med 2001;10:12–9.
12. Pennycott TW, Duncan G, Venugopal K. Marek's disease, candidiasis and megabacteriosis in a flock of chickens (*Gallus gallus domesticus*) and Japanese quail (Coturnix japonica). Vet Rec 2003;153:293–7.
13. Martins NR, Horta AC, Siqueira AM, et al. *Macrorhabdus ornithogaster* in ostrich, rhea, canary, zebra finch, free range chicken, turkey, guinea-fowl, columbina pigeon, toucan, chuckar partridge and experimental infection in chicken, Japanese quail and mice. Arq Bras De Med Vet Zootech 2006;58:291–8.
14. Jansson DS, Brojer C, Mattsson R, et al. *Mycotic proventriculitis* in gray partridges (*Perdix perdix*) on two game bird farms. J Zoo Wildl Med 2008;39:428–37.
15. Hanka K, Koehler K, Kaleta EF, et al. *Macrorhabdus ornithogaster*: detection in companion birds, poultry and pigeons, morphological characterisation and examination of in vitro cultivation. Prakt Tierarzt 2010;91:390–5.
16. Piasecki T, Prochowska S, Celmer Z, et al. Occurrence of *Macrorhabdus ornithogaster* in exotic and wild birds in Poland. Med Weter 2012;68:245–9.
17. Phalen DN. Diagnosis and management of *Macrorhabdus ornithogaster* (formerly megabacteria). Vet Clin Exot Anim 2005;8:299–306.
18. Simpson VR. Megabacteriosis in exhibition budgerigars. Vet Rec 1992;131:203–4.
19. Fillippich LJ, Herdrikz JK. Prevalence of megabacteria in budgerigar colonies. Aust Vet J 1998;76:92–5.
20. Phalen DN, Hanafusa Y, Costa E, et al. Further investigation into the biology of Macrorhabdus ornithogaster. Association of Avian Veterinarians Australian Committee, Annual Conference, Melbourne (Victoria). Australia. August 9–11, 2005. p. 75–8.
21. Mutlu OF, Seckin S, Ravelhofer SK, et al. Proventriculitis in fowl caused by megabacteria. Tierarztl Prax 1997;25:460–2.
22. Schulze C, Heidrich R. Megabacteria-associated proventriculitis in poultry in the state of Brandenburg, Germany. Dtsch Tierarztl Wochenschr 2001;108:264–6.
23. Behnke EL, Fletcher OJ. *Macrorhabdus ornithogaster* (Megabacterium) infection in adult hobby chickens in North America. Avian Dis 2011;55:331–4.

24. Huchzermyer F, Henton NM. Megabacteria in mammals. Vet Rec 2000;146:768.
25. Cooke SW. Role of megabacteria in mammals. Vet Rec 2000;147:371–2.
26. Hanafusa Y, Costa E, Phalen DN. Infection trials in mice suggest that *Macrorhabdus ornithogaster* is not capable of growth in mammals. Med Mycol 2013;51: 669–72.
27. Baker JR. Clinical and pathological aspects of 'going light' in exhibition budgerigars (*Melopsittacus undulatus*). Vet Rec 1985;116:406–8.
28. Filippich LJ, Parker MG. Megabacteriosis and proventricular/ventricular disease in psittacines and passerines. In: Proceedings of the Annual Conference of the Association of Avian Veterinarians. Reno (NV): Association of Avian Veterinarians. September 28–30, 1994. p. 287–93.
29. Kheirandish R, Salehi M. Megabacteriosis in budgerigars: diagnosis and treatment. Comp Clin Pathol 2011;20:501–5.
30. Schmidt R, Reavell D, Phalen DN. Pathology of exotic birds. Ames (IA): IA Iowa State University Press; 2003.
31. Hanafusa Y, Bradley A, Tomaszewski EK, et al. Growth and metabolic characterization of *Macrorhabdus ornithogaster*. J Vet Med Diag 2007;19:256–65.
32. Phalen DN, Tomaszewski E, Davis A. Investigation into the detection, treatment, and pathogenicity of avian gastric yeast. In: Proceedings of the 23rd Annual Conference of the Association of Avian Veterinarians. Monterey (CA): Association of Avian Veterinarians. August 26–30, 2002. p. 49–51.
33. Filippich LJ, Perry RA. Drug trials against megabacteria in budgerigars (*Melopsittacus undulatus*). Aust Vet Pract 1993;23:184–9.
34. Gestier AW. Treatment of megabacteria in budgerigars by in water medication with soluble amphotericin B. Available at: http://www.vetafarMcoMau/pages/Megabacteria-in-Australian-Budgerigars.html. Accessed October 1, 2014.
35. Bradley A, Yasuka H, Phalen DN. *Macrorhabdus ornithogaster*: inhibitory drugs, oxygen toxicity and culturing from feces. USDA sponsored summer research program Athens (GA), July 26–28, 2005.
36. Hoppes S. Treatment of *Macrorhabdus ornithogaster* with sodium benzoate in budgerigars (*Melopsittacus undulates*). In: Proceedings of the 23rd Annual Conference of the Association of Avian Veterinarians. Seattle (WA): Association of Avian Veterinarians. August 11–15, 2012. p. 67.
37. Phalen DN, Moore R. Experimental infection of white-leghorn cockerels with *Macrorhabdus ornithogaster* (Megabacterium). Avian Dis 2003;47:254–60.

Raptor Gastroenterology

Maureen Murray, DVM, DABVP (Avian)

KEYWORDS

- Raptors • Rehabilitation • Gastrointestinal anatomy • Gastrointestinal physiology
- Nutrition • Gastrointestinal disease conditions

KEY POINTS

- Raptor gastrointestinal anatomy and physiology differ substantially from noncarnivorous birds.
- An understanding of raptor gastroenterology is crucial to the successful rehabilitation of free-living raptors.
- Providing proper nutrition and critical care nutritional support are imperative to gastrointestinal and overall health.
- Clinicians treating free-living raptors should be aware of infectious and noninfectious causes of gastrointestinal pathology.

Free-living raptors are frequently presented to wildlife rehabilitation centers, often due to anthropogenic factors, such as motor vehicle collisions and toxicoses.[1–3] Restoring these birds to health and returning them to the wild is both challenging and rewarding. A thorough understanding of the anatomy, physiology, and natural history of these species is crucial to successful treatment and rehabilitation. This article addresses raptor gastroenterology with an emphasis on conditions affecting free-living birds.

The term *raptor* encompasses a variety of avian species with different natural histories, anatomic features, and diets. Most commonly, *raptor* is used to refer to hawks, falcons, and owls. Although these birds share certain similarities, they are taxonomically distinct groups. Based on genetic analyses showing that birds in the family Falconidae are not closely related to other birds previously included in the order Falconiformes, in 2010 the American Ornithologists' Union (AOU) recognized the new order, Accipitriformes, which contains 3 families.[4] Owls are in the order Strigiformes, which contains 2 families. Current classification based on the AOU Checklist of North and Middle American Birds[5] is given in **Table 1**.

ANATOMY AND PHYSIOLOGY
Beak and Tongue

Raptors have strong, curved beaks, the color of which varies among species. In birds of the genus *Falco*, the beak is distinguished by a notch along the cutting

Disclosures: None.
Wildlife Clinic, Department of Infectious Disease and Global Health, Tufts Cummings School of Veterinary Medicine, 200 Westboro Road, North Grafton, MA 01536, USA
E-mail address: maureen.murray@tufts.edu

Vet Clin Exot Anim 17 (2014) 211–234
http://dx.doi.org/10.1016/j.cvex.2014.01.006
vetexotic.theclinics.com

Table 1
Current American Ornithologists' Union classification of raptors

Order	Family	Birds Included	Examples
Falconiformes	Falconidae	Falcons, caracaras	Peregrine falcon (*Falco peregrinus*), American kestrel (*Falco sparverius*)
Accipitriformes	Accipitridae	Hawks, eagles, kites	Red-tailed hawk (*Buteo jamaicensis*), bald eagle (*Haliaeetus leucocephalus*), Cooper's hawk (*Accipiter cooperii*)
	Pandionidae	Osprey	Osprey (*Pandion haliaetus*)
	Cathartidae	New World vultures	Turkey vulture (*Cathartes aura*), California condor (*Gymnogyps californianus*)
Strigiformes	Strigidae	Typical owls	Great horned owl (*Bubo virginianus*), eastern screech-owl (*Megascops asio*)
	Tytonidae	Barn owls	Barn owl (*Tyto alba*)

edge, or tomia, of the upper bill, referred to as the tomial tooth or tomial notch (**Fig. 1**). This structure is believed to allow falcons to quickly sever the spinal cord of their prey.[6]

Food is manipulated with the beak and tongue, which like in most other birds (except parrots) lacks intrinsic muscles.[7] The tongue in raptors is nonprotrusible, and the rostral portion is firm and rough.[7] In eagles and vultures, the rostral portion of the tongue may be curved into a troughlike shape (**Fig. 2**).[7]

Esophagus and Crop

The crop, or ingluvies, is an enlargement of the cervical esophagus that functions to store food,[8] allowing a bird to ingest a large amount to be digested at a later time. Spindle-shaped crops are present in the Falconiformes and Accipitriformes.[9] The crop is particularly well developed in vultures (**Fig. 3**).[10] The Strigiformes do not have crops,[9] but food can be stored throughout the length of the esophagus.[8]

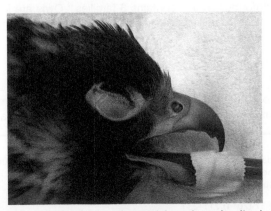

Fig. 1. An anesthetized peregrine falcon. The tomial notch on the distal aspect of the upper bill is a characteristic of birds in the genus *Falco*.

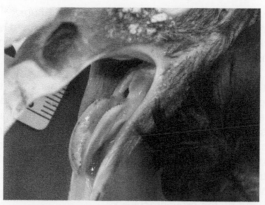

Fig. 2. The tongue of a turkey vulture, showing the characteristic troughlike shape seen in this species, as well as in eagles.

Proventriculus and Ventriculus (Gizzard)

Carnivorous and piscivorous birds possess an undifferentiated type of stomach, which differs significantly from the highly differentiated type seen in herbivores and granivores.[8] As in other birds, the raptor stomach is composed of the proventriculus (pars glandularis) and the ventriculus or gizzard (pars muscularis), with the proventriculus being the site of gastric juice secretion.[8,11] However, given the soft consistency of their diets, the raptor gizzard is not required to perform the degree of mechanical

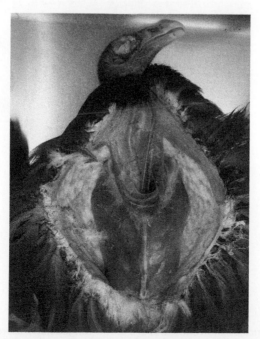

Fig. 3. A turkey vulture cadaver dissected to show the crop. Although small when empty, the crop is highly distensible and capable of storing a large amount of food.

digestion that occurs in birds consuming diets of a harder nature.[8,11] In contrast to the thick-walled gizzards of granivores, the carnivore/piscivore gizzard is thin-walled, relatively poorly muscled, and lacks the opposing pairs of thick and thin muscles that are responsible for the contractions that grind the food in many other avian species (**Fig. 4**).[8,9,11]

The proventriculus and gizzard of raptors serve as expandable storage organs to accommodate large prey items and as the site of chemical digestion.[8,11] Externally, there may be little obvious distinction between the proventriculus and gizzard.[8,11] The proventriculus is lined by mucosal ridges (plicae proventricularis) (**Fig. 5**), which are absent in noncarnivores and serve to increase the storage capacity of the proventriculus.[8] Gastric juice from the proventriculus maintains a low pH in the gizzard, which is the site of gastric proteolysis.[7] The cuticle, or koilin layer, which is produced by mucosal glands of the gizzard, functions primarily to protect the mucosa from the gastric juice produced by the proventriculus.[8,11]

Gastric Digestion and Pellet Egestion

The digestive process in raptors differs substantially from that in birds more commonly seen by veterinarians, such as psittacines. Because of the decreased need for mechanical grinding of food in raptors, the sequence of muscular contractions in the stomach is much simpler than the contraction sequence in species such as psittacines, which have paired thick and thin muscles in the gizzard.[7] In addition, indigestible components of the prey are retained in the gizzard, compacted into a pellet, and egested. The egestion of pellets, also referred to as *castings* in falconry terms, prevents indigestible material from passing through the entire gastrointestinal (GI) tract.[9]

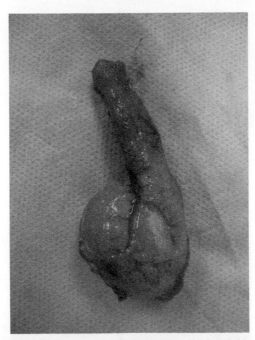

Fig. 4. The proventriculus and ventriculus of a broad-winged hawk (*Buteo platypterus*). The ventriculus in birds of prey is thin-walled compared with granivorous birds, as the raptor diet requires little mechanical digestion.

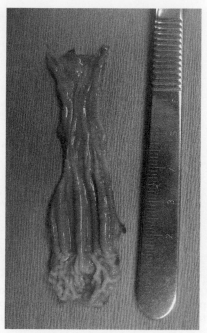

Fig. 5. The esophagus, proventriculus, and ventriculus of a Cooper's hawk showing the mucosal ridges (plicae proventricularis) in the proventriculus, which allow the proventriculus to expand to increase storage capacity.

Egestion is a process unique to birds, as it does not share the characteristics of emesis or regurgitation in mammals.[12]

Gastric digestion has been studied in great horned owls and is broken into the following 4 phases.[9]

1. Filling of the stomach: During this phase, muscular contractions in the proventriculus and gizzard are of high amplitude and moderate to high frequency.
2. Chemical digestion: A 4-hour to 8-hour period of low-amplitude, low-frequency muscular contractions.
3. Fluid evacuation: A 1-hour to 2-hour period of slowly increasing gastric contractions.
4. Pellet egestion: High-amplitude and high-frequency contractions occur in the gizzard for 4 to 10 minutes, followed by strong esophageal antiperistalsis, which causes pellet egestion. Movement of the pellet from the stomach to the mouth takes 8 to 12 seconds.

Pellet Composition

The composition of the pellet varies among groups of raptors; the pellets of some contain both hair and bones (eg, owls), whereas others contain predominantly hair (eg, hawks) (**Fig. 6**).[9] **Table 2** details the composition of pellets by taxonomic group.

A study that compared gastric digestion among 7 species of raptors found that the stomachs of birds in the families Falconidae and Accipitridae are significantly more acidic (pH 1.6) than the stomachs of birds in the family Strigidae (pH 2.35).[17] The more acidic gastric environment of the hawks, eagles, and falcons in the study is likely

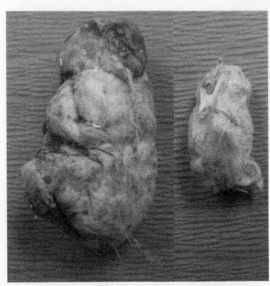

Fig. 6. Pellets from a red-tailed hawk (*left*) and an eastern screech-owl (*right*). A fragment of bone is visible in the owl pellet, whereas the hawk pellet consists predominantly of fur. The color of the pellets is characteristic of birds that are fed white laboratory mice in the rehabilitation setting.

the reason for the more complete digestion and bone corrosion in these birds compared with owls.[17]

Pellet Appearance and Frequency of Egestion

The appearance of the pellet varies with the diet. Raptors fed white laboratory mice will produce tan-colored pellets (see **Fig. 6**), whereas the pellet produced from a meal obtained in the wild is usually darker because of the color of the fur or feathers of the prey. Fresh pellets may be covered with mucus and occasionally some bile staining can be seen on the surface of a pellet. There should be no odor to the pellet.

It is important to monitor pellet egestion in raptors, as failure to produce a pellet can indicate dysfunction of GI tract. The frequency of pellet egestion varies with taxonomic group. Although multiple factors appear to influence the meal-to-pellet interval (MPI),[18–23] following are some general guidelines.

- Owls: Owls generally egest 1 pellet per meal. The stimulus appears to be the presence of the pellet in the gizzard.[22] Studies have shown that larger meals result in a longer MPI.[20,22,23] However, MPI also increased in barred owls (*Strix*

Table 2
Pellet composition by taxonomic group

Order	Family	Pellet Composition
Falconiformes	Falconidae	Predominantly hair[9]
Accipitriformes	Accipitridae	Predominantly hair[9]
	Pandionidae	Scales and bones[13]
	Cathartidae	Hair, vegetable matter, minimal to no bone[14–16]
Strigiformes	Strigidae	Hair and bone[9]
	Tytonidae	Hair and bone[9]

varia) fed a submaintenance compared with maintenance amount of food, indicating a potential ability to increase digestive time and thoroughness in response to nutritional needs.[20]

- Hawks and falcons: Hawks and falcons have been noted to egest 1 pellet per 2 to 3 meals, but also multiple pellets per 1 meal if meal size was large.[18,21,22] Some studies have found that hawks egest at dawn in response to photoperiod.[18,22] Although in another study, captive hawks fed late in the day did not cast at dawn; they did have shorter MPIs than hawks fed at dawn, supporting a potential role of photoperiod.[19] This response to photoperiod is suggested to be an adaptation to diurnal hunting, allowing the stomach to be empty during the time of day the bird is seeking prey.[19] Variation in pellet composition, size, and frequency based on the parts of the prey that are eaten has been noted.[18,21]
- Ospreys: Pellets are small and rarely seen, which indicates that most of their dietary items pass through the entire GI tract.[13]
- Vultures: Pellets are produced at unknown intervals.[14–16] In a rehabilitation setting, pellets may be difficult to discern if the bird exhibits regurgitation as a stress response when observed or handled.[22]

Small Intestine

The avian small intestine (SI) is shorter than in mammals.[11,24] There is less variation in the structure and function of the SI among birds than there is in the stomach,[10] although carnivorous birds have a shorter SI than granivorous birds, as the digestion of meat occurs more rapidly.[8,10,11] There are relative differences in SI length among raptors. Piscivores have longer SIs than meat eaters; vultures also have longer SIs relative to species that eat live prey; and birds that hunt other birds on the wing have shorter SIs than those that hunt by soaring or pouncing, which is likely an adaptation to decrease weight and increase agility in the air.[25] This difference in SI length affects digestive efficiency: a longer SI allows higher efficiency.[25] This subject is discussed further under "Nutrition."

As in other birds, the SI is the principal site of chemical digestion and nutrient absorption.[7,24] The villi in carnivores are better developed than in noncarnivorous birds, which compensates for the shorter length of the SI.[10] The SI consists of the duodenum, jejunum, and ileum, although there is little histologic differentiation among these regions, which are mainly demarcated by anatomic position.[8,10,11] The intestinal loops are arranged in various patterns dependent on species and are generally referred to with the following terminology:

- Duodenal loop: contains the pancreas[7]; tends to be elongated in hawks, falcons, and eagles.[8]
- Axial loop: contains Meckel's diverticulum, which is the remnant of the yolk sac and marks the junction between the jejunum and ileum; composed of both jejunum and ileum.[7]
- Supraduodenal loop: the most distal loop of the ileum, which is so named because it lies dorsal to the duodenum.[7]
- Supracecal loop: seen in only a few species of birds, including hawks, eagles, and falcons; composed of a section of the distal region of the ileum close to the ileo-rectal junction.[7,8]

Ceca

Birds have paired ceca that originate from the rectum at the junction of the rectum and the ileum.[10,24] Avian ceca are classified into 4 types: intestinal, glandular, lymphoid, and vestigial.[26] The Accipitriformes and Falconiformes have very small ceca of the lymphoid type.[27] Although small or vestigial ceca are generally characteristic of carnivorous birds, owls are an exception to this generality, as they have large ceca (**Fig. 7**).[10,24] Owls possess glandular ceca that contain goblet cells and secretory glands.[8,10,24]

The function of the ceca in owls is not well understood, although it has been hypothesized that they play a role in water balance.[28,29] In a study in which cecectomy was performed in great horned owls, no change in food metabolizability or in body weight was noted compared with control owls.[28] Although the cecectomized owls did show an initial increase in water consumption, by 21 days postoperatively water consumption had returned to normal.[28] However, a separate study that also performed cecectomy in great horned owls and then subjected them to heat stress found that the owls lost body mass and became dehydrated, indicating that the ceca likely do function to maintain water balance under certain environmental conditions.[29] In other raptors, water balance is entirely maintained by the kidneys and the rectum.[30]

Cecal contents are evacuated with less frequency than rectal feces.[11] Cecal droppings can be distinguished from rectal feces in that they are of a softer consistency, usually very dark in color,[11,24] and may be voluminous. Cecal droppings can be observed in owls periodically and should not be mistaken for diarrhea (**Fig. 8**).

Rectum

The rectum in birds is short and extends from the ileocecal junction to the cloaca.[24] American kestrels, however, have a relatively long rectum, which is thought to be particularly important in maintaining water balance in this species.[31] Histologically, the rectum is similar to the SI but has shorter villi.[24] The rectum opens into the coprodeum in the cloaca.

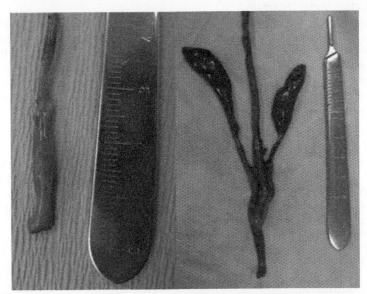

Fig. 7. The ceca of a Cooper's hawk (*left*) and a barred owl (*right*). Strigiformes differ from other carnivorous birds in that they have large ceca, which most likely play a role in water balance.

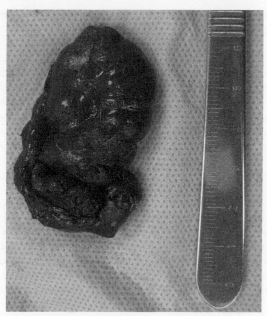

Fig. 8. A cecal dropping from a great horned owl. These droppings can be less formed than shown in this photograph and should not be mistaken for diarrhea.

Nearly continuous antiperistalsis occurs in the rectum, which is interrupted when defecation occurs.[24] This antiperistalsis moves urine and feces from the cloaca into the rectum, where water and sodium chloride are resorbed before excretion.[32] In owls, rectal antiperistalsis moves contents into the ceca.[24]

Appearance of the Feces

Thorough examination of the droppings (referred to as *mutes* in falconry terms) is essential to evaluating the GI tract. The appearance of the feces can vary based on the diet, but the feces should be formed and are generally dark brown in color and surrounded by white urates and a small amount of clear urine (**Fig. 9**). The feces may be tan colored in birds fed day-old chicks.[6,33] Watery feces can occur in birds that are not fed appropriate casting material.[34] Anorexia is a common cause of green feces due to

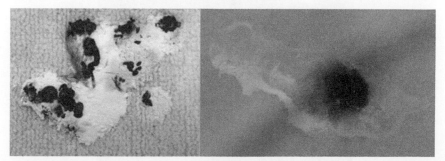

Fig. 9. Normal feces from a merlin (*Falco columbarius, left*) and green-colored feces from an anorexic bald eagle (*right*). The urine component of the dropping is not visible in these photographs.

the passage of bile. Some birds may intermittently have green feces unrelated to anorexia or underlying pathology.[34]

Liver and Pancreas

Although in many avian species the right lobe of the liver is larger than the left,[7] in raptors this size difference is less pronounced. Birds of prey possess gall bladders, which are located in the right lobe of the liver.[7] Carnivorous species have particularly well developed gall bladders (**Fig. 10**).[8] The avian pancreas has 3 lobes: dorsal, ventral, and splenic.[7] Pancreatic secretions are similar to mammals; amylase, lipase, and trypsin are produced.[7,8] In carnivores, the pancreas is relatively small, which is thought to be due to the high digestibility of the diet.[11,30]

NUTRITION

Proper nutrition is crucial to GI and overall health. It is essential to know the appropriate diet for a given species. Many falcons and birds in the genus *Accipiter* require avian prey. Ospreys are strictly fish-eaters. Although the diet of some species, such as barred owls and red-tailed hawks, is composed predominantly of small to medium-sized mammals, these birds also consume avian and amphibian prey. Some small raptors, such as American kestrels and eastern screech-owls, regularly consume insects.

Digestive Efficiency

Specialist feeders, such as birds in the genus *Accipiter* and falcons, have shorter SI lengths relative to other raptors.[8,10,11] Because of this decrease in SI length, these birds have decreased digestive efficiency compared with generalist feeders with longer SIs.[25] A study that compared the efficiency of digestion in a specialist feeder, the peregrine falcon, and a generalist, the common buzzard (*Buteo buteo*), found that when the 2 birds were fed the same diets, the peregrine falcon absorbed 7% less of the diet than the common buzzard.[25] Moreover, the peregrine falcon lost body mass when fed a mammalian prey item but gained body mass when fed an equivalent amount of an avian prey item.[25] Although the common buzzard gained body mass on both diets, it gained more when feeding on the avian diet.[25] These results suggest that some prey items may be more efficiently assimilated, possibly because of a difference in fat content, which would compensate for decreased digestive efficiency

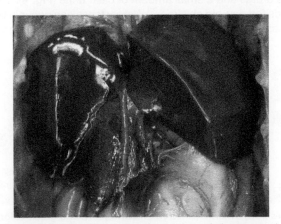

Fig. 10. The liver of a turkey vulture, showing the 2 lobes of almost equal size and the well-developed gall bladder.

in specialist feeders.[25] These results also stress the importance of feeding the appropriate diet for a given species.

Diet

Most raptors in a rehabilitation setting will readily eat dead prey if offered appropriate food items. Ospreys are a notable exception, and may require hand feeding during the length of the rehabilitation process.

The best diet to offer raptors in captivity is one that resembles the natural diet as closely as possible within the limitations of what food items are readily available and of high quality.[34–36] Food items should be obtained from a known and reputable source to prevent the possibility of disease transmission via the food and to ensure adequate nutrition of the prey items as well as humane handling of the animals.[36] Regular feeding of road kill should be avoided because of the potential presence of pathogens and toxins. Pigeons should not be fed to raptors, as several infectious diseases, including *Trichomonas gallinae* and herpesvirus, can be transmitted via this route.[6,34,37,38]

To ensure the diet is nutritionally balanced, it is crucial that whole prey items, including all internal organs, be offered to the bird.[31,35] It is also imperative that the food item be of appropriate size for the raptor to ensure the bird is able to consume the entire item.[36]

Because frozen/thawed items often lose some of their moisture content, soaking the items in water before feeding is often recommended.[6,34,36] Frozen/thawed fish are commonly fed to ospreys and bald eagles and must be supplemented with thiamine (30 mg/kg of fish as fed orally every 24 to 48 hours).[33,34,39] All raptors should have a fresh water source available at all times.

Allometric scaling, or determination of the daily minimum energy cost (MEC) can be used to determine the daily caloric needs for raptors in a rehabilitation setting.[40] The result of the equation $78 \times$ (body weight)$kg^{0.75}$ represents the minimum kilocalories (kcal) a bird of prey requires at rest. Using a simplistic but not grossly inaccurate assumption that 1 gram of prey item as fed equals 1 kcal, the result of this equation can be assumed to be the minimum amount of food (in grams) a raptor requires daily without taking into account potential increased needs for weight gain, activity, or healing. Although different vertebrate food items vary in their caloric content,[41] the assumption of 1:1 ratio can provide a reasonable, straightforward starting point for determining an amount to feed; however, birds should be weighed frequently and the amount fed adjusted as needed based on an individual bird's need for weight maintenance or gain.

Body condition can be assessed by palpation of pectoral muscle mass and visualization of subcutaneous fat stores. This physical evaluation of body condition should be used in conjunction with the body weight to determine a bird's nutritional requirements.

Common Food Items

Laboratory-raised or other captive-raised mice and/or rats, day-old chicks, and commercially available *Coturnix* quail are common food items used for raptors in a rehabilitation setting. In general, the nutritional composition of whole vertebrate prey is complete and fairly constant across types of prey items, differing mainly in the amount of fat present, which determines the caloric density.[31] The protein quality of vertebrate food items is excellent, as are the vitamin and mineral content and digestibility.[31,42–44] Laboratory-raised mice and rats tend to be higher in fat and lower in protein than free-living rodents, but overall they provide adequate nutrition to mammal-eating raptors.[36,44,45] Day-old chicks should be fed with the yolk sac intact[36,42] and, if fed to growing birds, calcium supplementation may be required.[42]

DISEASE CONDITIONS

Many infectious and noninfectious disease processes can affect the raptor GI tract. Highlighted as follows are select conditions with which clinicians treating free-living birds of prey should be familiar.

Parasitic

Trichomoniasis

Trichomoniasis, caused by the flagellated protozoan *T gallinae*, is the most clinically significant GI parasite of raptors.[6,46] In falconry terms, trichomoniasis is referred to as *frounce*. The main carriers of *T gallinae* are rock pigeons (*Columba livia*) and other columbiforms, such as mourning doves (*Zenaida macrourai*), in which species mortality events occasionally occur.[47] Virulent and avirulent strains of *T gallinae* exist.[47,48] Infection in raptors occurs after feeding on freshly killed infected prey. Young birds and adults that are debilitated due to other illness or injury are most susceptible.[37,49] Trichomoniasis has been seen in many species of raptors, including hawks, owls, and eagles.[6,47,50–52] Recent molecular analyses of *T gallinae* have characterized different strains of the organism.[51,53]

Studies of Cooper's hawks in Arizona found an association between prevalence of *T gallinae* in nestlings and proximity to urban environments.[54] Nestlings in an urban area showed 85% prevalence, whereas nestlings in a nonurban environment had 9% prevalence.[54] This difference is likely attributable to the higher numbers of mourning doves in the diets of urban hawks.[54] A separate study showed that mourning doves comprised 57% of the diet of urban hawks versus 4% of the diet in nonurban hawks.[55] Cooper's hawk nestlings in this same urban area had a 41% mortality rate attributed to trichomoniasis.[54]

T gallinae causes caseous plaques and granulomas that invade the mucosa of the oropharynx, crop, and esophagus, and can also involve the sinuses and trachea.[6,37] In severe cases, large granulomas can form that obstruct the esophagus and cause difficulty swallowing (**Fig. 11**). The granulomas can also cause dyspnea by impinging on the trachea and can destroy normal anatomic structures in the oropharynx, such as the choana.

Affected free-living birds present in poor body condition due to an inability to eat. The oral cavity may have a foul odor. Plaques or granulomas can be appreciated on oral examination or palpation of the esophagus and crop. In less-severe cases, birds may appear hungry but unable to eat. "Head flicking" behavior, or tearing off pieces of food and tossing them aside, may be observed.[6,37,46] Diagnosis can be made by swabbing the crop with a cotton-tipped applicator moistened with warm saline and examining a wet mount microscopically. The motile, flagellated protozoa can be observed using $\times 40$ magnification.

Carnidazole (30 mg/kg single oral dose[37] or repeated every 24 hours for 2–3 days[6]) is an effective and previously commonly used treatment; however, carnidazole is currently not available in the United States. Metronidazole (30–50 mg/kg orally every 24 hours for 3–5 days[6,37]) also can be used. In severe cases in which large granulomas or tissue destruction has occurred, prognosis is poor.[6] However, successful treatment of severe cases in captive falcons with metronidazole at 100 mg/kg orally every 24 hours for 3 days, followed by surgical removal of granulomas 3 to 7 days after metronidazole therapy has been reported.[56]

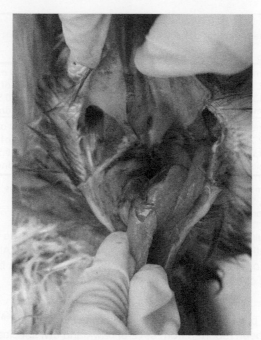

Fig. 11. The oral cavity of a red-tailed hawk, partially dissected to show a large granuloma caused by *Trichomonas gallinae*. The granuloma can be seen at the base of the tongue and also extended into the cervical esophagus.

Helminths

In free-living birds of prey, intestinal parasites are commonplace and in most circumstances do not cause clinical disease. In young birds and in debilitated or injured adults further stressed by the process of rehabilitation, however, clinical signs are more likely to occur, and treatment is warranted, as high parasite loads can have negative effects. Clinical signs of intestinal parasitism are nonspecific and generally include anorexia, weight loss, and diarrhea. Free-living birds of prey in a rehabilitation setting that will not self-feed or that present in poor body condition should be checked for parasites and treated accordingly. Studies in free-living hawks, falcons, owls, eagles, and ospreys have found that the most common parasites in these birds are nematodes and trematodes.[57–61] Antiparasitics for the treatment of helminths are given in **Table 3**.

Capillaria spp are the most commonly encountered nematode in raptors.[6,37,46,62] Most species of capillarids have a direct life cycle, although some use earthworms as intermediate hosts.[63] Low levels of infection are frequent in free-living birds and do not cause clinical signs; however, heavy infection can result in illness.[63] *Capillaria* can occur in the oropharynx and throughout the GI tract. The oropharyngeal form causes caseous oral plaques, which can resemble trichomoniasis. Diagnosis is by oral swab, which may reveal the bioperculate ova characteristic of *Capillaria* spp. A high intestinal *Capillaria* load can cause diarrhea, anorexia, and weight loss. Ova will be seen on fecal flotation.

Ascarids are common in free-living raptors, including *Porrocaecum* spp and *Contracaecum* spp.[6,46,62] Ascarids can occur in the small intestine, proventriculus, and gizzard, and cause disease if high numbers of worms are present.[6,46,62] Life cycles can be direct or indirect depending on species.[46,62] *Contracaecum* spp are particularly common in fish-eating birds.[64] Characteristic roundworm ova will be seen on fecal flotation.

Table 3
Antiparasitics for the treatment of helminths

Helminth	Drug	Dose
Nematodes	Drontal Plus (22.7 mg praziquantel, 22.7 mg pyrantel pamoate, 113.4 mg febantel)[a]	0.0064 × MEC[b] PO once (result implies the proportion of the tablet to administer; eg, 0.5 = $\frac{1}{2}$ tablet)
	Ivermectin	0.2–0.4 mg/kg SC once[65]
Trematodes	Drontal Plus (22.7 mg praziquantel, 22.7 mg pyrantel pamoate, 113.4 mg febantel)[a]	0.0064 × MEC[b] PO once (result implies the proportion of the tablet to administer; eg, 0.5 = $\frac{1}{2}$ tablet)
	Praziquantel	10 mg/kg PO, SC once, repeat in 7 d[65]

Abbreviations: MEC, minimum energy cost; PO, by mouth; SC, subcutaneous.
[a] Bayer HealthCare, Shawnee Mission, KS.
[b] See "Nutrition" for explanation of MEC calculation.

Trematodes require several intermediate hosts and usually reside in the small intestine, although infections of the bile ducts and liver can occur.[49,62] Although infections are usually asymptomatic, severe liver pathology and death have been reported.[6,49] Large, operculated ova will be seen on fecal flotation.

Coccidia

Free-living birds of prey may carry coccidia without clinical signs.[66] Eimeria and Caryospora spp have been reported from several hawk and owl species.[67,68] To date, 15 species of Caryospora have been identified from free-living raptors.[69] Recently, new species of Caryospora have been identified from a sharp-shinned hawk (Accipiter striatus)[69] and a bald eagle.[70]

Coccidia in free-living birds likely occur in low numbers and do not cause pathology in healthy individuals, but can be pathogenic in individuals that are stressed or debilitated or that ingest large numbers of oocyts.[67] Death of a free-living juvenile Eurasian kestrel (Falco tinnunculus) that demonstrated weakness, emaciation, and hemorrhagic enteritis due to Caryospora spp infection has been reported.[71]

Treatment options include sulfadimethoxine 50 mg/kg orally once, then 25 mg/kg orally every 24 hours for 3 to 7 days[65] or toltrazuril 10 mg/kg orally every 24 hours for 2 days, repeat in 14 days.[6]

Viral

Herpesvirus

Herpesvirus infections in birds of prey cause hepatic necrosis and death. Previously, herpesviruses were categorized as falconid herpesvirus 1 (FHV-1) and strigid herpesvirus 1 (StHV-1).[72] Transmission of the virus to raptors has long been recognized as being via consumption of pigeons.[6,38] Recent genetic analysis has determined that FHV-1 and StHV-1 are identical to columbid herpesvirus 1 (CoHV-1), which causes disease in squabs and is carried subclinically by adult pigeons.[72] Since this discovery, CoHV-1 has been identified in free-living great horned owls and Cooper's hawks in North America, as well as in 2 species of native Australian owls and 1 native Australian falcon.[72–75]

Reported antemortem signs include acute onset of anorexia and vomiting.[72,75] Disease progression is rapid, with death usually occurring within 48 hours of infection.[38] Characteristic gross postmortem lesions include enlarged liver and spleen, with multifocal tan or white nodules.[72–75] Hemorrhage within the intestinal tract may be seen.[75] On histopathologic examination, hepatic, splenic, and intestinal necrosis will be seen.[72-75] Eosinophilic intranuclear inclusion bodies may be seen in liver, spleen, intestine, bone marrow, and possibly other tissue.[72-75] Diagnosis can be confirmed by polymerase chain reaction. Prevention of herpesvirus infection in raptors in a captive setting entails avoiding feeding pigeons.

Adenovirus

Adenoviruses cause hepatitis and enteritis, which can result in mortality, particularly in young birds. Most reports describe infections in falcon species.[76-79] Adenovirus antibodies have been detected in free-living common buzzards,[80] and recently an adenovirus has been isolated from free-living black kites (*Milvus migrans*).[81] Molecular analysis of an adenovirus isolated from an outbreak in a raptor propagation and reintroduction facility that primarily affected neonatal northern aplomado falcons (*Falco femoralis septentrionalis*) was found to belong to the genus *Aviadenovirus*.[76,77]

Adenoviruses are spread via a fecal-oral route and possibly via inhalation.[6] Although previously the route of transmission was believed to have possibly been via infected prey, it has now been shown in falcons that certain species, particularly peregrine falcons, can be asymptomatic carriers of adenoviruses that can act as primary pathogens in other species.[76,77] Additionally, a fatal case in a free-living American kestrel that was trapped for research purposes may have been precipitated by the stress of handling and captivity, suggesting that latent infection may cause disease under certain conditions.[78]

Sudden death may occur with no antemortem signs. When clinical signs are observed, they include anorexia, lethargy, and hemorrhagic diarrhea.[77,82-85] Characteristic lesions on histopathologic examination included hepatic necrosis with basophilic intranuclear inclusion bodies within hepatocytes and possibly other tissues, including spleen and intestines.[77,78]

Treatment consists of supportive care, and the prognosis is grave. Prevention in rehabilitation centers should focus on not cohousing different species of falcons.[76,77] Adenoviruses are resistant to many disinfectants, including chlorhexidine; quaternary ammonium compounds are among the agents recommended for poultry adenoviruses.[82]

Toxic

Lead

Lead toxicosis is the most significant toxicant that affects the GI tract in raptors. All raptor species are susceptible; however, those that scavenge on large prey items or waterfowl that contain fragments of lead ammunition are most at risk of exposure.[86-88] Commonly affected species in North America include bald eagles, golden eagles (*Aquila chrysaetos*), and California condors. Lead poisoning contributed to the near extinction of the California condor and remains a barrier to reestablishment of the population.[89]

Along with affecting the erythropoietic system and the central nervous system, lead poisoning affects the motility of the GI tract. GI-related signs of lead poisoning include crop stasis, ileus, diarrhea, and regurgitation.

Lead particles may be, but are not always, detected in the gizzard on radiographs (**Fig. 12**). Diagnosis is by determination of blood lead level through a commercial laboratory or an in-house analyzer (LeadCare II Blood Lead Testing System; Magellan Diagnostics, North Billerica, MA). There are species differences among raptors in sensitivity to lead, with turkey vultures and condors more resistant relative to other species.[90,91] Eagles with blood lead levels higher than 100 μg/dL (1.00 ppm) are

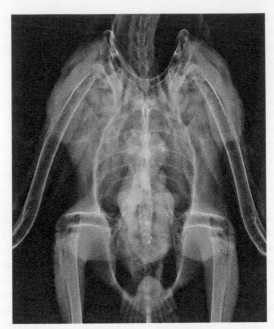

Fig. 12. Radiograph of a turkey vulture showing lead fragments in the gizzard.

reported to have a poor prognosis for recovery[88,92]; however, successful treatment of California condors with blood lead levels of 200 µg/dL (2.9 ppm)[91] and 440 µg/dL (4.4 ppm)[93] have been documented. In general, a blood lead level of 20 µg/dL (0.2 ppm) or higher should prompt treatment, as levels higher than this value are considered to be above background exposure.[6,88,92]

Use of the chelators Calcium-EDTA (CaEDTA; 30–50 mg/kg every 12 hours subcutaneously or intramuscularly) and dimercaptosuccinic acid (DMSA; 30–40 mg/kg orally every 12 hours) have been reported in raptors.[6,91–95] DMSA is very effective at decreasing blood lead levels and removing lead from soft tissue but will not chelate lead bound in bone, whereas CaEDTA very effectively removes lead stored in bone.[92] Because of these differences, combination therapy has been recommended and is likely more effective than single therapy with either chelator, particularly in severely affected birds.[92]

Protocols regarding length of therapy vary.[92] A 3-day to 5-day course of chelation followed by 2 to 3 days off chelation has often been recommended based on protocols used in children.[92] Repeated blood lead measurement then guides the need for further treatment. CaEDTA has a wide margin of safety in birds,[94] and more prolonged therapy (up to 3 weeks) and doses of up to 100 mg/kg have been reported with no adverse effects.[92] DMSA may have a narrower margin of safety and careful dosing may be warranted.[94] Continuous therapy with DMSA for up to 10 days without adverse effects has been reported in several species of zoo birds.[95]

Additional treatment includes general supportive care, and removal of lead present in the GI tract by means of endoscopy, gavage, or surgery when patient condition allows. Use of promotility agents, such as metoclopromide, has been recommended.[92] However, promotility agents were not effective in resolving crop stasis in California condors with lead toxicosis.[91,93] Ingluviostomy tubes have been used successfully in the management of crop stasis in California condors.[91,93]

Starvation

Raptors can present in a state of starvation for several reasons; for example, adult birds that have been nonflighted and unable to hunt because of an injury; young-of-the-year that are not yet adept hunters; or birds that become trapped in a building or other human-made structure. A thorough evaluation for chronic injuries that may result in the bird being nonreleasable, including a complete ophthalmic examination, should be performed in all emaciated raptors.

Free-living birds of prey face periods of food shortage under natural conditions because of severe weather or decreased prey availability, and several studies on fasting in raptors have been conducted to elucidate the metabolic changes that occur.[96–98] Findings from these studies are summarized as follows:

- A study in common buzzards found these birds to be tolerant of complete food deprivation for 13 days. Although the birds lost 26% of their initial body mass and showed evidence of catabolizing body protein for energy, with unrestricted refeeding, all birds regained lost mass. No significant changes in hematocrit or total protein were seen during the fasting phase.[96]
- A study in barn owls showed that these birds withstood complete food deprivation for 8 days and were able to restore lost body mass within 8 days of unrestricted refeeding. Increased tissue protein utilization was observed. The birds lost an average of 28% of body mass during the fasting phase of the study, but were still able to fly and self-feed when food was reintroduced. However, this same study examined emaciated owls that had been killed by motor vehicle collisions and found evidence that although emaciated birds could still fly, their ability to digest food appeared to be impaired.[97]
- A study in American kestrels showed that when completely deprived of food for 3 days, these birds showed decreased metabolism, decreased body temperature, and lost 17% to 20% of body mass. Although all birds recovered and regained 11% of body mass within 24 hours of ad libitum refeeding, the investigators concluded that American kestrels would likely die of starvation if completely deprived of food for 5 days.[98]

These studies show that the species of raptors examined are tolerant of acute food deprivation for varying amounts of time, with smaller species tolerant for a shorter period than larger species. These controlled experiments do not mimic conditions of decreased food intake over a more prolonged period of time, however.

In determining a treatment plan for a chronically malnourished raptor in the rehabilitation setting, parallels are often drawn to refeeding syndrome in human medicine, which refers to a condition that occurs in malnourished patients after enteral or parenteral nutrition is provided.[99,100] Refeeding syndrome can occur in people who have had minimal food intake for 5 days or longer.[99] During starvation in people, protein and fat become the main energy sources instead of carbohydrates.[99,100] Refeeding syndrome in people is characterized by shifts in fluids and electrolytes that occur following increased insulin and decreased glucagon secretion in response to the sudden availability of nutrients, including glucose, as the body switches from a catabolic to an anabolic state.[99,100] The result of these electrolyte shifts can be a fatal hypophosphatemia, hypokalemia, and hypomagnesemia.[99,100]

Glucose metabolism in birds of prey is different from humans, as well as from granivorous birds, given that their diet is high in protein and lipid and low in carbohydrate.[101,102] Studies indicate that birds have lower insulin and higher glucagon levels compared with mammals[101,103] and that carnivorous birds have lower insulin levels compared with chickens.[101] It appears that glucagon rather than insulin is the main hormone regulating glucose metabolism in birds.[103,104] Studies in barn owls and black vultures (*Coragyps atratus*) have found that in both fasting and fed states these species exhibit a high rate of gluconeogenesis using amino acids to maintain blood glucose (BG)[101,102,105] and that BG is resistant to prolonged fasting because of this high rate of gluconeogenesis.[102,105]

Because of these metabolic differences, it is difficult to draw exact comparisons between the pathophysiology of refeeding syndrome in people to physiologic derangements that may occur in chronically malnourished raptors. However, nutritional support for emaciated raptors in the rehabilitation setting should be approached carefully. Severe anemia and hypoproteinemia are hematological changes that may identify a chronically malnourished raptor.[6,106,107]

Protocols for treating falconry birds in low condition (ie, at a critically low body weight) have been described[6,33,34,106] and are likely applicable to the free-living raptor. Guidelines for treating a chronically malnourished raptor include the following:

- Provide heat to prevent the bird from expending energy on thermoregulation.
- Normalize hydration status over 12 to 24 hours before offering nutrition.
  - Subcutaneous fluids are an effective route of administration.
  - Be mindful of the risk of fluid overload if the intravenous or intraosseous routes are used.
  - Continue fluid support for 3 to 5 days after feeding is reinstituted.
- Supplement with thiamine and other B vitamins before and during initial refeeding; this may be warranted because of their role in energy metabolism (B vitamin complex dosed at 1–2 mg/kg of thiamine subcutaneously every 24 hours).
- Introduce small volumes/amounts of easily digestible food divided into 3 to 4 feedings per day.
  - Critical care feeding formulas (eg, Iams Maximum-Calorie [The Iams Company, Cincinnati OH], Emeraid Carnivore [Lafeber Company, Cornell, IL]) can be used, if available, and delivered via gavage feeding for 1 to 2 days.
  - Formulas should be warmed and diluted initially with water or an isotonic electrolyte solution.
  - Initial volume (in milliliters) should be approximately 3% of body weight (in grams).
  - Concentration and/or volume of the solution (not to exceed 5% of body weight) can be increased with each feeding if tolerated.
- Introduce whole prey items devoid of fur or feathers, soaked in warm water.
  - Feed small amounts (one-fourth MEC total initially) divided into 3 to 4 feedings per day (see "Nutrition" section for description of MEC calculation).
  - Incrementally increase the total daily amount by one-fourth MEC each day until the bird is eating at least 2 MEC to promote weight gain.
  - Introduce casting material when the bird is eating 1 MEC, provided the bird is passing normal feces.
- Perform a fecal examination for intestinal parasites in all birds presented in an emaciated state and administer an antiparasitic as indicated.

During refeeding in humans, careful monitoring and supplementation of phosphorous, potassium, calcium, and magnesium is recommended,[99,100] but is generally impractical in a wildlife rehabilitation setting. As there are currently no documented cases describing the pathophysiology of a refeeding-like syndrome in free-living raptors, a practical approach to chronically malnourished birds should focus on incremental introduction of high-quality nutrition suitable for strict carnivores (high protein, high fat, minimal carbohydrates).

SUMMARY

In summary, conditions affecting the raptor GI tract can be the primary reason for a free-living bird of prey to be presented to a wildlife rehabilitation center, or the GI tract may be affected secondarily as a result of debilitation from other injuries or the stress of the rehabilitation process. Successful rehabilitation and release of raptors requires thorough evaluation of and attention to the entire bird. Knowledge of raptor gastroenterology and nutrition is crucial to restoring and maintaining the health of the bird during rehabilitation and to returning a healthy raptor to its natural environment.

REFERENCES

1. Harris MC, Sleeman JM. Morbidity and mortality of bald eagles (*Haliaeetus leucocephalus*) and peregrine falcons (*Falco peregrinus*) admitted to the Wildlife Center of Virginia, 1993-2003. J Zoo Wildl Med 2007;38:62–6.
2. Wendell MD, Sleeman JM, Kratz G. Retrospective study of morbidity and mortality of raptors admitted to Colorado State University Veterinary Teaching Hospital during 1995 to 1998. J Wildl Dis 2002;38:101–6.
3. Deem SL, Terrell SP, Forrester DJ. A retrospective study of morbidity and mortality of raptors in Florida: 1988–1994. J Zoo Wildl Med 1998;29:160–4.
4. Chesser RG, Banks RC, Barker FK, et al. Fifty-first supplement to the American Ornithologists' Union Check-List of North and Middle American Birds. Auk 2010; 127.726–44.
5. American Ornithologists' Union. AOU checklist of North and Middle American birds. Available at: http://checklist.aou.org/taxa. Accessed September 3, 2013.
6. Redig PT, Cruz-Martinez L. Raptors. In: Tully TN, Dorrestein GM, Jones AK, editors. Handbook of avian medicine. 2nd edition. New York: Saunders Elsevier; 2009. p. 209–42.
7. King AS, McLelland J. Digestive system. In: Birds: their structure and function. 2nd edition. London: Bailliere Tindall; 1984. p. 84–109.
8. McLelland J. Digestive system. In: King AS, McLelland J, editors. Form and function in birds, vol. 1. London: Academic Press; 1979. p. 69–181.
9. Duke GE. Gastrointestinal physiology and nutrition in wild birds. Proc Nutr Soc 1997;56:1049–56.
10. Klasing KC. Anatomy and physiology of the digestive system. In: Comparative avian nutrition. New York: CABI Publishing; 1998. p. 9–35.
11. Denbow DM. Gastrointestinal anatomy and physiology. In: Whittow GC, editor. Sturkie's avian physiology. 5th edition. San Diego (CA): Academic Press; 2000. p. 299–325.
12. Duke GE, Evanson OA, Redig PT, et al. Mechanism of pellet egestion in great-horned owls (*Bubo virginianus*). Am J Physiol 1976;231:1824–9.
13. Poole AF. Diet and foraging ecology. In: Ospreys: a natural and unnatural history. Cambridge (United Kingdom): Cambridge University Press; 1989. p. 67–84.
14. Kirk DA, Mossman MJ. Turkey vulture (*Cathartes aura*). In: Poole A, Gill F, editors. The birds of North America, No. 339. Philadelphia: The Birds of North America, Inc; 1998. p. 1–32.
15. Snyder NF, Schmitt NJ. California condor (*Gymnogyps californianus*). In: Poole A, Gill F, editors. The birds of North America, No. 610. Philadelphia: The Birds of North America, Inc; 2002. p. 1–36.

16. Buckley NJ. Black vulture (*Coragyps atratus*). In: Poole A, Gill F, editors. The birds of North America, No. 411. Philadelphia: The Birds of North America, Inc; 1999. p. 1–24.
17. Duke GE, Jegers AA, Loff G, et al. Gastric digestion in some raptors. Comp Biochem Physiol 1975;50A:649–56.
18. Balgooyen TG. Pellet regurgitation by captive sparrow hawks (*Falco sparverius*). Condor 1971;73:382–5.
19. Fuller MR, Duke GE, Eskedahl DL. Regulation of pellet egestion: the influence of feeding time and soundproof conditions on meal to pellet intervals of red-tailed hawks. Comp Biochem Physiol 1979;62A:433–8.
20. Duke GE, Fuller MR, Huberty BJ. The influence of hunger on meal to pellet intervals in barred owls. Comp Biochem Physiol 1980;66A:203–7.
21. Duke GE, Tereick AL, Reynhout JK, et al. Variability among individual American kestrels (*Falco sparverius*) in parts of day-old chicks eaten, pellet size, and pellet egestion frequency. J Raptor Res 1996;30:213–8.
22. Duke GE, Evanson OA, Jegers A. Meal to pellet intervals in 14 species of captive raptors. Comp Biochem Physiol 1976;53A:1–6.
23. Kostuch TE, Duke GE. Gastric motility in great horned owls (*Bubo virginianus*). Comp Biochem Physiol 1975;51A:201–5.
24. Duke GE. Alimentary canal: anatomy, regulation of feeding, and motility. In: Sturkie PD, editor. Avian physiology. 4th edition. New York: Springer-Verlag; 1986. p. 269–88.
25. Barton NW, Houston DC. A comparison of digestive efficiency in birds of prey. Ibis 1993;135:363–71.
26. Clench MH, Mathias JR. The avian cecum: a review. Wilson Bull 1995;107:93–121.
27. Clench MH. The avian cecum: update and motility review. J Exp Zool 1999;283: 441–7.
28. Duke GE, Bird JE, Daniels KA, et al. Food metabolizability and water balance in intact and cecectomized great-horned owls. Comp biochem physiol 1981;68A: 237–40.
29. Chaplin SB. Effect of cecectomy on water and nutrient absorption of birds. J Exp Zool Suppl 1989;3:81–6.
30. Klasing KC. Digestion of food. In: Comparative avian nutrition. New York: CABI Publishing; 1998. p. 36–70.
31. Klasing KC. Nutritional strategies and adaptations. In: Comparative avian nutrition. New York: CABI Publishing; 1998. p. 71–124.
32. Johnson OW. Urinary organs. In: King AS, McLelland J, editors. Form and function in birds, vol. 1. London: Academic Press; 1979. p. 183–235.
33. Joseph V. Raptor medicine: an approach to wild, falconry, and educational birds of prey. Vet Clin North Am Exot Anim Pract 2006;9:321–45.
34. Cooper JE. Nutritional diseases, including poisoning, in captive birds. In: Birds of prey: health and disease. 3rd edition. Oxford: Blackwell Science Ltd; 2002. p. 143–62.
35. Heidenreich M. Feeding. In: Birds of prey: medicine and management. Oxford: Blackwell Science Ltd; 1997. p. 24–34.
36. Chitty J. Raptors: nutrition. In: Chitty J, Lierz M, editors. BSAVA manual of raptors, pigeons, and passerine birds. 2nd edition. Gloucester (MA): British Small Animal Veterinary Association; 2008. p. 190–201.
37. Forbes NA. Raptors: parasitic diseases. In: Chitty J, Lierz M, editors. BSAVA manual of raptors, pigeons, and passerine birds. 2nd edition. Gloucester (MA): British Small Animal Veterinary Association; 2008. p. 202–11.

38. Stanford M. Raptors: infectious diseases. In: Chitty J, Lierz M, editors. BSAVA manual of raptors, pigeons, and passerine birds. 2nd edition. Gloucester (MA): British Small Animal Veterinary Association; 2008. p. 212–22.
39. Carpenter JW. Nutritional/mineral support used in birds. In: Exotic animal formulary. 4th edition. St Louis (MO): Elsevier Saunders; 2013. p. 302–8.
40. Pokras MA, Karas M, Kirkwood JK, et al. An introduction to allometric scaling and its uses in raptor medicine. In: Redig PT, Cooper JE, Remple D, et al, editors. Raptor biomedicine. Minneapolis (MN): University of Minnesota Press; 1993. p. 211–24.
41. Dierenfeld ES, Alcorn HL, Jacobsen KL. Nutrient composition of whole vertebrate prey (excluding fish) fed in zoos. Nat Agric Libr Z7994, Z65, p. 20. Available at: http://www.nal.usda.gov/awic/zoo/WholePreyFinal02May29.pdf. Accessed February 13, 2014.
42. Bird DM, Ho SK. Nutritive values of whole-animal diets for captive birds of prey. Raptor Res 1976;10:45–9.
43. Tabaka CS, Ullrey DE, Sikarskie JG, et al. Diet, cast composition, and energy and nutrient intake of red-tailed hawks (*Buteo jamaicensis*), great horned owls (*Bubo virginianus*), and turkey vultures (*Cathartes aura*). J Zoo Wildl Med 1996;27:187–96.
44. Douglas TC, Pennino M, Dierenfeld ES. Vitamins E and A, and proximate composition of whole mice and rats used as feed. Comp Biochem Physiol 1994;107A:419–24.
45. Crissey SD, Slifka KA, Lintzenich BA. Whole body cholesterol, fat, and fatty acid concentrations of mice (*Mus domesticus*) used as a food source. J Zoo Wildl Med 1999;30:222–7.
46. Cooper JE. Parasitic diseases. In: Birds of prey: health and disease. 3rd edition. Oxford (United Kingdom): Blackwell Science Ltd; 2002. p. 105–20.
47. U.S. Geological Survey. Trichomoniasis. In: Friend M, Franson JC, editors. Field manual of wildlife diseases: general field procedures and diseases of birds. Madison (WI): USGS Biological Resources Division; 1999. p. 201–6.
48. Forrester DJ, Foster GW. Trichomoniasis. In: Atkinson CT, Thomas NJ, Hunter DB, editors. Parasitic diseases of wild birds. Ames (IA): Wiley-Blackwell; 2008. p. 120–53.
49. Heidenreich M. Parasitic diseases. In: Birds of prey: medicine and management. Oxford (United Kingdom): Blackwell Science Ltd; 1997. p. 131–52.
50. Ueblacker SN. Trichomoniasis in American kestrels (*Falco sparverius*) and eastern screech-owls (*Otus asio*). In: Lumeij JT, Remple JD, Redig PT, et al, editors. Raptor biomedicine III. Lake Worth (FL): Zoological Education Network; 2000. p. 59–63.
51. Sansano-Maestre J, Garijo-Toledo MM, Gomez-Munoz MT. Prevalence and genotyping of *Trichomonas gallinae* in pigeons and birds of prey. Avian Pathol 2009; 38:201–7.
52. Stone WB, Nye PE. Trichomoniasis in bald eagles. Wilson Bull 1981;93:109.
53. Gerhold RW, Yabsley MJ, Smith AJ, et al. Molecular characterization of the *Trichomonas gallinae* morphologic complex in the United States. J Parasitol 2008;94:1335–41.
54. Boal CW, Mannan RW, Hudelson KS. Trichomoniasis in Cooper's hawks from Arizona. J Wildl Dis 1998;34:590–3.
55. Estes WA, Mannan RW. Feeding behavior in Cooper's hawks at urban and rural nests in southeastern Arizona. Condor 2003;105:107–16.
56. Samour JH, Naldo JL. Diagnosis and therapeutic management of trichomoniasis in falcons in Saudi Arabia. J Avian Med Surg 2003;17:136–43.

57. Kinsella JM, Cole RA, Forrester DJ, et al. Helminth parasites of the osprey, *Pandion haliaetus*, in North America. J Helm Soc Wash 1996;63:262–5.

58. Kinsella JM, Foster GW, Cole RA, et al. Helminth parasites of the bald eagle, *Haliaeetus leucocephalus*, in Florida. J Helm Soc Wash 1998;65:65–8.

59. Kinsella JM, Foster GW, Forrester DJ. Parasitic helminths of five species of owls from Florida USA. Comp Parasitol 2001;68:130–4.

60. Richardson DJ, Kinsella JM. New host distribution records for gastrointestinal parasites of raptors from Connecticut, USA. Comp Parasitol 2010;77:72–82.

61. Baker DG, Morishita TY, Bartlett JL, et al. Survey of internal parasites of northern California raptors. J Zoo Wildl Med 1996;27:358–63.

62. Smith SA. Parasites of birds of prey: their diagnosis and treatment. Sem Avian Exotic Pet Med 1996;5:97–105.

63. Yabsley MJ. Capillarid nematodes. In: Atkinson CT, Thomas NJ, Hunter DB, editors. Parasitic diseases of wild birds. Ames (IA): Wiley-Blackwell; 2008. p. 463–97.

64. Fagerholm HP, Overstreet RM. Ascaridoid nematodes: Contracaecum, Porrocaecum, and Baylisascaris. In: Atkinson CT, Thomas NJ, Hunter DB, editors. Parasitic diseases of wild birds. Ames (IA): Wiley-Blackwell; 2008. p. 413–33.

65. Carpenter JW. Antiparasitic agents used in birds. In: Exotic animal formulary. 4th edition. St Louis (MO): Elsevier Saunders; 2013. p. 229–55.

66. U.S. Geological Survey. Intestinal coccidiosis. In: Friend M, Franson JC, editors. Field manual of wildlife diseases: general field procedures and diseases of birds. Madison (WI): USGS Biological Resources Division; 1999. p. 207–13.

67. Upton SJ, Campbell TW, Weigel M, et al. The Eimeriidae (Apicomplexa) of raptors: review of the literature and description of new species of the genera *Caryospora* and *Eimeria*. Can J Zool 1990;68:1256–65.

68. Lindsay DS, Blagburn BL. *Caryospora uptoni* and *Frenkelia* sp.-like coccidial infections in red-tailed hawks (*Buteo borealis*). J Wildl Dis 1989;25:407–9.

69. McAllister CT, Duszynski DW, McKown RD. A new species of *Caryospora* (Apicomplexa: Eimeriidae) from the sharp-shinned hawk, *Accipiter striatus* (Aves: Accipitriformes). J Parasitol 2013;99:490–2.

70. McAllister CT, Duszynski DW, McKown RD. A new species of *Caryospora* (Apicomplexa: Eimeriidae) from the bald eagle, *Haliaeetus leucocephalus* (Accipitriformes: Accipitridae), from Kansas. J Parasitol 2013;99:287–9.

71. Krone O. Fatal *Caryospora* infection in a free-living juvenile Eurasian kestrel (*Falco tinnunculus*). J Raptor Res 2002;36:84–6.

72. Gailbreath KL, Oaks JL. Herpesviral inclusion body disease in owls and falcons in caused by the pigeon herpesvirus (Columbid herpesvirus 1). J Wildl Dis 2008; 44:427–33.

73. Pinkerton ME, Wellehan JF, Johnson AJ, et al. Columbid herpesvirus-1 in two Cooper's hawks (*Accipiter cooperii*) with fatal inclusion body disease. J Wildl Dis 2008;44:622–8.

74. Rose N, Warren AL, Whiteside D, et al. Columbid herpesvirus-1 mortality in great horned owls (*Bubo virginianus*) from Calgary, Alberta. Can Vet J 2012; 53:265–8.

75. Phalen DN, Holz P, Rasmussen L, et al. Fatal columbid herpesvirus-1 infections in three species of Australian birds of prey. Aust Vet J 2011;89:193–6.

76. Oaks JL, Schrenzel M, Rideout B, et al. Isolation and epidemiology of falcon adenovirus. J Clin Microbiol 2005;43:3414–20.

77. Schrenzel M, Oaks JL, Rotstein D, et al. Characterization of a new species of adenovirus in falcons. J Clin Microbiol 2005;43:3402–13.

78. Tomaszewski EK, Phalen DN. Falcon adenovirus in an American kestrel (*Falco sparverius*). J Avian Med Surg 2007;21:135–9.
79. Schelling SH, Garlick DS, Alroy J. Adenoviral hepatitis in a merlin (*Falco columbaris*). Vet Pathol 1989;26:529.
80. Frolich K, Prusas C, Schettler E. Antibodies to adenoviruses in free-living common buzzards from Germany. J Wildl Dis 2002;38:633–6.
81. Kumar R, Kumar V, Asthana M, et al. Isolation and identification of a fowl adenovirus from wild black kites (*Milvus migrans*). J Wildl Dis 2010;46:272–6.
82. Dean J, Latimer KS, Oaks JL, et al. Falcon adenovirus infection in breeding Taita falcons (*Falco fasciinucha*). J Vet Diagn Invest 2006;18:282–6.
83. Forbes NA, Simpson GN, Higgins RT, et al. Adenovirus infection in Mauritius kestrels (*Falco punctatus*). J Avian Med Surg 1997;11:31–3.
84. Van Wettere AJ, Wunschmann A, Latimer KS, et al. Adenovirus infection in Taita falcons (*Falco fasciinucha*). J Avian Med Surg 2005;19:280–5.
85. Zsivanovits P, Monks DJ, Forbes NA. Presumptive identification of a novel adenovirus in a Harris hawk (*Parabuteo unicinctus*), a Bengal eagle owl (*Bubo bengalensis*), and a Verreauzx's eagle owl (*Bubo lacteus*). J Avian Med Surg 2006;20:105–12.
86. Kelly TR, Johnson CK. Lead exposure in free-flying turkey vultures is associated with big game hunting in California. PLoS One 2011;6:e15350.
87. Kelly TR, Bloom PH, Torres SG. Impact of the California lead ammunition ban on reducing lead exposure in golden eagles and turkey vultures. PLoS One 2011;6: e17656.
88. Stauber E, Finch N, Talcott PA. Lead poisoning of bald (*Haliaeetus leucocephalus*) and golden (*Aquila chrysaetos*) eagles in the US inland Pacific Northwest region—an 18-year retrospective study: 1991-2008. J Avian Med Surg 2010; 24:279–87.
89. Finkelstein ME, Doak DF, George D, et al. Lead poisoning and the deceptive recovery of the critically endangered California condor. Proc Natl Acad Sci U S A 2012;109:11449–54.
90. Carpenter JW, Pattee OH, Fritts SH, et al. Experimental lead poisoning in turkey vultures (*Cathartes aura*). J Wildl Dis 2003;39:96–104.
91. Wynne J, Stringfield C. Treatment of lead toxicity and crop stasis in a California condor (*Gymnogyps californianus*). J Zoo Wildl Med 2007;38:588–90.
92. Redig PT, Arent LR. Raptor toxicology. Vet Clin North Am Exot Anim Pract 2008; 11:261–82.
93. Aguilar RF, Yoshicedo JN, Parish CN. Ingluviotomy tube placement for lead-induced crop stasis in the California condor (*Gymnogyps californianus*). J Avian Med Surg 2012;26:176–81.
94. Denver MC, Tell LA, Galey FD, et al. Comparison of two heavy metal chelators for treatment of lead toxicosis in cockatiels. Am J Vet Res 2006;61:935–40.
95. Hoogesteijn A, Raphael BL, Calle P, et al. Oral treatment of avian lead intoxication with meso-2,3-dimercaptosuccinic acid. J Zoo Wildl Med 2003;34: 82–7.
96. Garcia-Rodriguez T, Ferrer M, Carrillo JC, et al. Metabolic responses of *Buteo buteo* to long-term fasting and refeeding. Comp Biochem Physiol 1987;87A: 381–6.
97. Handrich Y, Nicholas L, Le Maho Y. Winter starvation in captive common barn-owls: physiological states and reversible limits. Auk 1993;110:458–69.
98. Shapiro CJ, Weathers WW. Metabolic and behavioral responses of American kestrels to food deprivation. Comp Biochem Physiol 1981;68A:111–4.

99. Mehanna HM, Moledina J, Travis J. Refeeding syndrome: what it is, and how to prevent and treat it. BMJ 2008;336:1495–8.
100. Stanga Z, Brunner A, Leuenberger M, et al. Nutrition in clinical practice—the refeeding syndrome: illustrative cases and guidelines for prevention and treatment. Eur J Clin Nutr 2008;62:687–94.
101. Myers MR, Klasing KC. Low glucokinase activity and high rates of gluconeogenesis contribute to hyperglycemia in barn owls (Tyto alba) after a glucose challenge. J Nutr 1999;129:1896–904.
102. Migliorini RH, Linder C, Moura JL, et al. Gluconeogenesis in a carnivorous bird (black vulture). Am J Physiol 1973;225:1389–92.
103. Braun EJ, Sweazea KL. Glucose regulation in birds. Comp Biochem Physiol 2008;151B:1–9.
104. Hazelwood RL. Pancreas. In: Whittow GC, editor. Sturkie's avian physiology. 5th edition. San Diego (CA): Academic Press; 2000. p. 539–55.
105. Veiga JA, Roselino ES, Migliorini RH. Fasting, adrenalectomy, and gluconeogenesis in the chicken and a carnivorous bird. Am J Physiol 1978;234:R115–21.
106. Redig PT. Nursing avian patients. In: Beynon PH, editor. BSAVA manual of raptors, pigeons, and waterfowl. Gloucestershire (MA): British Small Animal Veterinary Association Limited; 1996. p. 42–6.
107. Smith EE. Haematologic parameters on various species of Strigiformes and Falconiformes. J Wildl Dis 1978;14:447–50.

Diet and Its Role in the Behavioral Health and Training of Exotic Species

Barbara Heidenreich, BS Zoology

KEYWORDS

- Positive reinforcement • Behavior problems • Reinforcers • Food preference
- Motivation • Food management • Primary reinforcers • Secondary reinforcers

KEY POINTS

- Food plays a significant role in influencing animal behavior.
- Avian and small mammal species show general trends in food preferences that can be used for reinforcing desired behaviors.
- Motivation for food can be increased by various strategies.
- Nonfood reinforcers offer options for reinforcing behaviors when food is of little value.
- Transitioning to healthier diets can help prevent reproductive hormone amplification in companion parrots, which can make undesired behavior more easily triggered.

 Video of guinea pig motivated to climb onto a scale; aviary birds motivated for training; managed delivery of a skunk's regular diet; Macaw with free access to pelleted food; and a rabbit calm and relaxed for nail trimming accompany this article at http://www.vetexotic.theclinics.com/

POSITIVE REINFORCEMENT TRAINING

Science-based behavior-change technology is becoming an integral part of the management of many companion animal species, including exotics. This technology uses the least intrusive principles as defined by behavior analysis to influence animal behavior to address behavioral problems, manage husbandry, reduce or eliminate stress for routine medical care, and preserve the human-animal bond.

To effectively train new behaviors and maintain a relationship based on trust with an animal, conscientious trainers focus on using positive reinforcement. Reinforcement is the procedure of providing consequences for a behavior that increases or maintains

Good Bird Inc, PO Box 150604, Austin, TX 78715, USA
E-mail address: Barb@GoodBirdInc.com

Vet Clin Exot Anim 17 (2014) 235–247
http://dx.doi.org/10.1016/j.cvex.2014.01.007
1094-9194/14/$ – see front matter © 2014 Elsevier Inc. All rights reserved.

the frequency of that behavior.[1] Positive reinforcement indicates that something is added to the environment to increase or maintain the designated behavior. In animal training, positive reinforcers tend to be things the animal seeks to acquire or values, and may include preferred food items, access to enrichment items, tactile, companionship, and, in some cases, verbal responses from caregivers.[2]

FOOD AS A REINFORCER

Consequences that serve to increase or maintain a behavior are called reinforcers,[3] both primary and secondary. A primary reinforcer is defined as a reinforcing stimulus that has acquired its properties as a function of species history.[4] In general, primary reinforcers are often described as essential to life. Secondary reinforcers are those that depend on their association with other reinforcers, and are also known as conditioned reinforcers.[4]

Food is a primary reinforcer. Under certain circumstances food has the potential to be a powerful reinforcer, which can make it a very useful tool in influencing animal behavior. In some animal training communities, using food to reinforce behavior is viewed as failure or inappropriate. However, when reviewing the natural history of animals and how consequences are always influencing animal behavior, it becomes clear that using food to reinforce behavior is expanding on a natural process that is already occurring.

In the wild and in captivity, animals frequently enact behaviors to acquire food. This behavior may be as simple as walking from point A to point B to feed from a bowl, to presenting complex foraging behaviors that require an animal to express its adaptations for feeding, to participating in a structured training session. Researchers have coined the term contrafreeloading to describe the phenomenon whereby animals choose to perform a learned response to obtain reinforcers, even when the same reinforcers are freely available.[5]

Food can be an exceptional tool in reinforcing behavior when conditions may not be supportive of the use of secondary reinforcers. For example, an animal that has no prior history with a caregiver may not be receptive to secondary reinforcers such as attention or tactile stimuli delivered from that individual. The animal may also not demonstrate a level of comfort that would allow it to engage in play activities in the presence of the person. In these situations food can be an excellent option for reinforcing acceptable behavior, and also associates desired consequences with the presence of the new person. This scenario can change the dynamic of the relationship between the animal and the trainer often much more quickly than not using food. This concept can also be applied to other objects or circumstances that may elicit a fear response in animals, such as items associated with restraint or the presence of unfamiliar items.[6]

Once food is accepted as a positive reinforcer, it also allows the trainer to pair food with other potential reinforcers to increase the list of desired consequences available for that animal. Food can be used to reinforce interacting with enrichment items, accepting tactile stimuli, and even accepting other food items as reinforcers.[6]

When food is considered a training tool, it can also open the door to noncoercive training strategies. For example, some trainers rely on jesses to maintain the behavior of sitting on the hand with bird species such as toucans, corvids, and kookaburras. Although the use of jesses is a practice historically used for raptor species, it has the potential to present health risks to bird species with delicate legs. Jesses use negative reinforcement to create the behavior of sitting on the hand. Allowing the use of food to train the behavior of sitting on the hand for a period of time gives a trainer the opportunity to focus on using positive reinforcement techniques, and avoid the potential injury that can be caused to nonraptor species wearing jesses.[7]

Another advantage to using food to reinforce behavior is the creation of a situation whereby an animal can quickly learn a new behavior. For example, during a 20-minute training session a trainer may have the opportunity to reinforce steps toward the desired behavior numerous times. Each repetition becomes a learning opportunity for the animal. A parrot can learn an entire behavior (such as step up on the hand, lift a foot, step onto a scale, accept fluid from a syringe) in a single training session when food is offered as a positive reinforcer and the bird is receptive to eating.[6]

Reinforcers differ between species and individuals. A list of food items commonly preferred by various species is given in **Table 1**.

In many cases the preferred food item toward which the animal gravitates needs to be monitored. Excessive amounts for some species or individuals may result in health problems, so it may be necessary to limit quantities. Other helpful strategies include using the smallest piece the animal will accept to reinforce behavior, allowing sufficient time to pass between training sessions, and using a variety of food and nonfood reinforcers when possible.

Table 2 presents a list of food items commonly preferred by various parrot species. This list is not exhaustive, and many individuals will respond to other food types as reinforcers. It is recommended that food items listed as preferred food items for reinforcing the behavior of parrots should be removed from the shell and broken into small pieces, although this does not apply to millet spray, safflower seed, and sunflower seeds in the shell. The recommended size to use for reinforcing desired behavior is one-third of a sunflower seed. Increasing or decreasing the size of the food item will depend on the species, level of motivation for food, and training strategy. In general, caregivers will have more opportunities to reinforce behavior if food items are kept small.

MOTIVATION FOR FOOD

Most trainers initiate a training session by assessing the animal's interest in the food that is available. The level of interest will determine whether to continue with a training session at that time. To better gauge acceptable levels of motivation, trainers define a range of observable behaviors that can be matched with levels of motivation for food. For example, when a pine nut is offered to a macaw in a training scenario where the bird is relaxed and comfortable and being asked to do nothing but accept food, the following observations could be used to rate motivation (**Table 3**).[2]

For most situations a medium level of interest in food is sufficient to create desired responses. Working with an animal with a low level of interest in food can create training problems such as slow response to the cue. Excessive levels of motivation often can result in less learning, as the animal is too focused on trying to acquire food. Both extremes are not ideal for animal training.[2]

When training a new behavior, it is generally advised to use the most preferred reinforcer. Once the behavior has transitioned to maintenance it can be advantageous to include other reinforcers, which can include a mix of food and nonfood reinforcers. This variety and unpredictability of which reinforcer will be offered can serve to maintain motivation for the animal to present the behavior.[2]

Motivation for reinforcers can be influenced by many conditions, including the environment. An important goal is for the animal to be relaxed and comfortable in the training area. For example, an animal that prefers to be in enclosed areas, such as a rat or guinea pig, may quickly climb onto a scale if a shelter is provided on the scale.

Table 1
Preferred food reinforcers for small mammals

Food Item	Rabbit	Guinea Pig	Rat	Hamster	Gerbil	Mouse	Chinchilla	Ferret
Greens	✔	✔						
Parsley	✔	✔						
Cilantro	✔	✔						
Carrots	✔ F	✔ F						
Apple	✔	✔						
Broccoli	✔							
Cantaloupe	✔	✔						
Watermelon	✔	✔						
Blueberries	✔							
Brussels sprouts	✔							
Grape							✔	
Raisin							✔	
Sunflower seeds			✔	✔	✔	✔		
Pumpkin seeds					✔			
Safflower seeds								
Millet spray	✔				✔	✔		
Peanuts				✔	✔	✔		
Pine nuts						✔		
Almonds					✔			
Pecans					✔			
Walnuts					✔			
Peanut butter			✔			✔		
Cooked butternut squash			✔ F					
Peas (thawed)			✔ F					
Pea organic natural baby food			✔					
Carrot organic natural baby food	✔							
Winter squash organic natural baby food			✔					
Plain oat cereal (eg, Cheerios)	✔ F							
Dried unsulfured papaya	✔ F							
Cooked meats								✔
Freeze-dried meats								✔
Meat-flavored organic baby food (low carb)								✔
Egg								✔

Abbreviation: F, favored.
Data from Heidenreich BE. Small mammal training. In: Proceedings Association of Avian Veterinarians. Association of Avian Veterinarians; 2012.

Table 2
Preferred food reinforcers for parrots

Food Item	Comments
Sunflower seeds in the shell: low oil preferred	Some parrots do not recognize shelled sunflower seeds
Shelled sunflower seeds	Preferred by many parrot species
Almond pieces	Preferred by many parrot species
Walnut pieces	Preferred by some individual parrots
Pistachio pieces	Preferred by some individual parrots
Pine nuts	Preferred by many larger parrot species
Millet spray	Preferred by many smaller parrot species. Conure sized and smaller. Of the large parrots, eclectus species often respond to millet
Macadamia pieces	Preferred by hyacinth macaws
Safflower seeds	These bitter seeds are often preferred by parrots in the genus *Poicephalus* and some conures
Unsulfured papaya bits	Moluccan and umbrella cockatoos and some Amazon parrots often respond to this food item
Peanut pieces	Preferred by many parrot species
Nectar, grape, apple	Preferred by lories and lorikeets

An overturned box with an access hole or hut on the scale can be tared out before the animal enters the shelter (Video 1).[2]

Other animals may respond with a higher level of comfort if a preferred companion is also in the training area. Some parrots and small mammals show behaviors that indicate discomfort when separated from conspecifics. The companion animal can be

Table 3
Assessing interest in reinforcers. Example: Macaw is offered a pine nut

Observed Behaviors	Level of Motivation
Holds pine nut in foot	Low
Bites tiny pieces off of pine nut slowly	Low
Drops half of the nut	Low
Wipes beak on perch (feaking observed)	Low
Proceeds to preen after drops nut	Low
Holds pine nut in foot and brings to mouth quickly	Medium
Quickly breaks nut into 2–3 pieces and swallows pieces	Medium
Directs attention back to trainer once nut is consumed	Medium
Swallows nut immediately without breaking into pieces	High
Quickly directs attention to trainer once nut is consumed	High
Offers trained behaviors in rapid succession	High
Presents behaviors equated with frustration or anxiety about food: may redirect aggressive behavior on nearby objects, birds, or people	Excessive
Aggressive behavior presented toward other birds if competing for the same food resource	Excessive

reinforced for remaining calm in the training area while the target animal is trained. Careful attention to arranging the environment to increase the comfort level of the animal in training will make it more likely that the animal will respond to available reinforcers.[2]

Trainers also aim for making it as easy as possible for the animal to present the behavior and acquire the reinforcer. For example, any behavior whereby the animal must physically move more to perform the action increases the difficulty, meaning that the animal must have higher motivation for the reinforcers provided. If the action is more easily accomplished by moving or adjusting props, it will require less motivation. For example, training a parrot to climb over the lip of a crate to walk into it is more difficult than walking directly into the transport container that is flush with the surface on which the bird is standing (**Fig. 1**).[2]

FOOD MANAGEMENT

If the animal is not interested in food, several strategies may be used by trainers to create motivation for food. For example, animals can be trained immediately preceding normal meal times, meal times can be staggered throughout the day to increase training opportunities, base diets can be provided at all times while preferred foods are saved for reinforcers to be offered during training, animals can be fed until satiation during training sessions several times a day, small pieces of food can be offered to allow for more repetitions before satiation, or caregivers can avoid overfeeding.[6] The following are examples whereby such strategies have proved to be successful in creating motivation for food reinforcers without compromising the health and welfare of the animal.

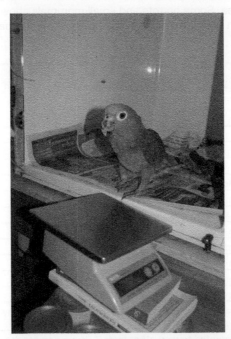

Fig. 1. Placing the scale so that it is flush with the floor and steady makes it easier for a parrot to step onto it, thus reducing the level of motivation for food required to obtain the behavior.

Train Just Before a Regularly Scheduled Feeding Time

In this strategy animals are fed a diet that is typically more than they can eat in a day. However, the diet may be removed for a period of time, for example, overnight. In the moments just before receiving a fresh supply of food, often animals are motivated to eat and can participate in a training session. This action can then be followed by the regular feeding.

Example. A mixed-species aviary that feeds from communal bowls normally received its daily feedings at 8:00 AM. At 7:30 AM training sessions for entering travel cages and standing on a scale were successfully conducted for food items normally received in the diet. The birds continued to have access to free amounts of food throughout day. At 5:00 PM uneaten food was discarded (Video 2).

Manage the Delivery of the Regular Diet

The amount and type of food the animal receives is not altered. Instead of presenting the full diet at one feeding time, the diet is offered in portions throughout the day in training sessions. By the end of the day the bulk or all of the diet should have been offered to the animal.

Example. A skunk at a wildlife facility was receiving a measured diet presented in a bowl at 5:00 PM each night. The empty bowl was removed in the morning. Motivation for food was created by taking that same diet and offering portions of it during training sessions throughout the day. Any food not used during the training session was offered to the skunk at the end of the last training session. The skunk received the entire diet daily. However, the skunk's behavior changed dramatically. Before managing the delivery of the diet the skunk was usually sleeping whenever keepers approached. After managing the delivery of the diet and embarking on a training program, the skunk was often waiting at the door in apparent anticipation of the training session. In addition, the skunk readily consumed portions of the diet offered during the training session. The skunk was trained to present a chained behavior of walking from a kennel to a bowl of dirt, digging in dirt, walking to a bag of garbage, digging in the garbage, and walking into a kennel to be presented for educational outreach programs (Video 3).

Free Feed a Base Diet and Reserve Preferred Food Items for Training Sessions

This strategy allows an animal access to food at all times. The motivation for food derives from the desire to gain the preferred food items during the training sessions.

Example. Parrots at a sanctuary had a pelleted diet in their bowl at all times. The birds received peanuts, sunflower seeds, fruit, and vegetables during training sessions. In a collection of 50 psittacines, every bird responded strongly to the food items offered during training. A blue and gold macaw was trained to voluntarily participate in nebulization using this feeding strategy (Video 4).[8]

Feed Until Satiated Each Training Session

This strategy involves using the animal's diet during a training session. The training session continues as long as the animal is willing to eat. When the animal shows signs of satiation, the session is ended and no more food is offered. Several more sessions are conducted wherein again the animal eats until satiated. No more food is offered at the end of the day. The animal's weight and response to food in each session can be monitored to help identify the appropriate number of training sessions per day.

Example. A mink at a wildlife rehabilitation facility was offered pieces of mice during training sessions. Although the mink was eager to participate, eventually the mink would begin to cache pieces of meat in the training area. The mink would continue to present behavior for food that it would then cache. However, the caching behavior was taken as an indication of satiation. The sessions were ended at the sign of repeated caching behavior. Two sessions per day allowed the mink to eat until satiated, and maintain a relatively stable body weight and response to food during training sessions. The mink was trained to target, enter a kennel, step on a scale, allow touching, allow a harnessing, and present a short chained behavior of hopping on a stump and running across a log.

Use Small Pieces of Food

A common practice in the companion animal community is the use of large pieces of food to reinforce behavior. Unfortunately, using food items that are very large can quickly satiate an animal. Although a large food item may help communicate that a particular response is more desirable than another, in general using the smallest food item an animal is willing to accept can allow a trainer many more opportunities to reinforce desired behavior.

Example. A companion parrot owner with a sun conure wanted to train her parrot to step up onto her hand without biting. The bird's preferred food reinforcer was goldfish crackers. Early in the training the owner was offering an entire goldfish cracker for approximations toward the desired behavior. After 2 repetitions and 2 crackers, the bird was satiated and no longer had an interest in the training session. For the next session the owner broke the cracker into tiny pieces. The bird progressed through all the approximations to the desired goal behavior in one session and consumed one cracker in the process.

Avoid Overfeeding

Overfeeding is a common contributor to health problems in companion animals, and can also interfere with achieving training goals. An animal with continual access to an overabundance of food is very unlikely to show a response to food items when offered, this can include preferred food items. Identifying and feeding an appropriate daily diet to maintain a healthy body mass for a companion animal can help increase motivation for a food (**Fig. 2**). This motivation can also lead to animals eating the entire diet,

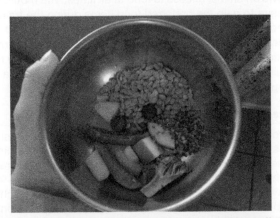

Fig. 2. An appropriate measured daily amount of food for a 550-g yellow-naped Amazon parrot (*Amazona auropalliata*).

including healthier elements that may be less palatable. One way caregivers can determine an appropriate daily amount is to measure the current diet before offering it, and measure the amount left over after access for 24 hours. This routine includes measuring items that may have been dropped or removed from the food bowl by the animal. This procedure can be applied for several days to determine an average amount of food consumed on a daily basis. This amount can then be offered as the daily diet. This amount may need to increase or decrease after a period of time depending on the animal's response to food when offered. Caregivers will also want to monitor the animal's weight to ensure sufficient amounts of food are supplied to maintain a healthy body mass when transitioning to a measured diet.

Example. An imprinted great horned owl received an excessive diet for several years. The bird would selectively eat only the preferred elements of the diet and routinely left behind large amounts of food. During the breeding season the bird presented aggressive behavior related to territory and nesting toward keepers and handlers. The owl also weighed 500 g more than the average for the species. Reducing the amount of food in the daily diet to an amount the bird could consume in a day allowed the owl to maintain a healthier body weight, eliminated the aggressive behavior, and made it possible for the bird to transition to a training program consequent to an increased interest in food as a reinforcer. The owl now readily participates as an ambassador bird for a zoo education program.

NONFOOD REINFORCERS

A primary reinforcer is a reinforcer whose effectiveness does not depend on its contingent relation to another reinforcer; this can be a stimulus, such as food, water, or sexual activity, that usually is reinforcing in the absence of any prior learning history. Such reinforcers are sometimes described as those necessary for the survival of the species.[4] The list of primary reinforcers is typically very small.

Secondary reinforcers are those that depend on their association with other reinforcers, also termed conditioned reinforcers, which consist of a stimulus that initially has no reinforcing properties but, through occurring simultaneously with unconditioned or strongly conditioned reinforcers, acquires reinforcing properties; they are also called learned reinforcers.[4] The list of secondary reinforcers can be endless. To distinguish between diet-related reinforcers and all others, the terms food and nonfood reinforcers are used in this article.

The power and role of nonfood reinforcers are often underestimated. Traditionally food has been the reinforcer of choice in training animals. Although this primary reinforcer can be extremely useful, nonfood reinforcers have proved to be valuable when animals are satiated on food reinforcers. In addition, including nonfood reinforcers in training can also help increase motivation by increasing reinforcer variety and allowing for novelty in reinforcers. This practice also provides a reinforcer that may retain its reinforcing value for long periods before an animal is satiated. By including nonfood reinforcers in the repertoire, trainers may find alternative means to influence behavior that can be very powerful.[9]

One obvious application of the use of nonfood reinforcers is when motivation for food reinforcers is low. One option is to consider means to create a higher level of motivation for food reinforcers, as described previously. Yet another option is to perform a reinforcer assessment to create a long list of other experiences, items, or circumstances that result in reinforcement without the use of food. The following are some examples in which nonfood reinforcers were used to maintain or increase desired behavior.

Contact with a Preferred Person as a Reinforcer

At a zoologic facility, contact with a preferred person was used as a reinforcer to train a conure to step up onto new people. This goal was achieved by having the preferred person place the bird on a table and step away. For this non flighted bird to have contact with the preferred person, the conure would step up onto a new person. The new person would then offer the bird the opportunity to step onto the preferred person. This action reinforced the behavior of stepping up onto a new person. Over time, staff members were able to phase out using the preferred person as the reinforcer.

Tactile as a Reinforcer

Many rabbits respond favorably to stroking from the nose toward the back of the head. A house rabbit was trained to present the behavior of digging on cue, which was reinforced by stroking on the head. Because of the rabbit's receptive response to touch, stroking was also paired with nail-trimming procedures. By pairing touch on the head with this process, nail trimming was accomplished without restraint. In addition, the rabbit presented calm, relaxed behavior throughout the procedure (Video 5).

Scent as Reinforcer

Mammal species often respond well to scent as a reinforcer. A male tamandua that was used in education programs was required to receive a generous diet to address a medical condition, which often led to food reinforcers having less value in training. However, the scent of a female tamandua and vinegar proved to be powerful reinforcers for this animal. Both have been used to reinforce behaviors such as climbing on a branch during presentations and returning to a kennel when cued.

Excitement/Toys as a Reinforcer

Parrots housed in an interactive aviary presented a problem behavior of flying into the guest entry-way to perch and chew on ceiling fans. To address this behavior, keepers looked for behaviors that typically preceded the problem behavior. In this case, the birds would often perch on a specific rope in anticipation of the door to the entry-way opening. When keepers noticed the conures on this perch, they cued the birds to fly to the hand. Once on the hand the birds were offered various small parrot-safe toys to destroy. Because the reinforcer for going to the entry-way was opportunities to chew other items, it was deemed that enrichment items/toys were the preferred reinforcer for the undesirable behavior and could be used to reinforce the acceptable behavior of flying to the hand.

FOOD AND BEHAVIOR

Food can play an interesting role in behavior. Some animals can learn to present aggressive behavior in the presence of food. This aggression is more commonly seen when resources are limited and competition for food resources exist or are perceived. In these situations, an animal may bite or lunge toward another animal or human that is attempting access to a food resource or food container. This behavior can persist once learned, even if food is abundant. In situations such as these, science-based behavior-change technology can be applied to teach the animal calm behavior toward others in the presence of food.

Animals that present aggressive behavior related to territory may also lunge, bite, and so forth when caregivers reach into a cage to access food bowls. This hostility can be addressed by teaching animals that waiting calmly will result in reinforcement.

Another alternative is to shift an animal into another enclosure or area, so that bowls are accessed when the animal is not present.

For parrots, the content and quantity of the diet also has the potential to influence behavior. In general a high-fat, high-carbohydrate diet paired with other environmental triggers can cause reproductive hormone amplification. This state often causes a parrot to be more easily triggered for aggressive behavior. It also encourages mate-seeking behavior, which can result in intense bonding with one person in the household and aggressive behavior toward others, cavity-seeking behavior and defense of these perceived nest sites, increased destructive behavior, and loud demanding vocalizations when left unattended. These behaviors are typically undesired by companion parrot owners, and can be avoided in part by preventing hormone amplification through provision of a less rich diet and appropriate quantity.[10]

TRANSITIONING AVIAN SPECIES TO PELLETED DIETS AND FRESH FOODS

Critical periods of development are specific times during which the environment has its greatest impact on an individual's development. This period has been studied extensively in dogs (and humans).[11] Anecdotally, critical periods of development are also observed in other animals. For many young animals, receptiveness to new experiences is observed during these times. For example, a young parrot may allow

Table 4	
Strategies to introduce parrots to pelleted diets and fresh foods	
Introducing Pellets	**Introducing Fresh Foods**
Soak pellets and roll dough into small balls. Roll balls in seed mixture. Over time reduce the amount of seeds and add hard pellets to dough	Weave fresh fruit and vegetables through cage bars
Sprinkle tiny pellets or crushed pellets over a wet-type food such as fresh fruit, vegetables, or mash	Insert fresh fruits and vegetables into foraging toys
Offer a 90% seed to 10% pellet ratio. Gradually reverse the percentages	Place seeds in bottom of bowl and cover with wet fresh fruit and vegetable
Prepare a bread or muffin using whole grains or pulverized pellets as flour. Mix seeds into the batter before baking	Sprinkle seeds on top of a mash that includes fresh fruits and vegetables
Insert pellets into foraging toys	Spread a soft food such as a fruit puree over seed mix
Soak pellets to create a mash and mix in seeds.	Insert partially visible seeds into pieces of fresh fruit and vegetables
Insert pellets into pieces of fresh fruit and vegetables	
Mix pellets into a pureed fruit or vegetables	
Introducing Both Pellets and Fresh Foods	
Let parrot view other birds eating the items	
Let parrot view a human eating the items	
Offer fresh foods and pellets in the morning and seed a few hours later	

For additional resources see the following articles available online:

The layered salad mix with instructions for diet conversion by Pamela Clark, CVT. Available at: http://www.pamelaclarkonline.com/Articles.html.

Diet conversion for seed junkie birds in food for different pet avian species by M. Scott Echols, DVM, Diplomate ABVP (Avian). Available at: http://www.avianstudios.com/wp-content/uploads/Foods-for-Different-Avian-Species3.pdf.

manipulation of its wings, feet, and beak. It may reach out to explore a nail file, towel, or new toy. It may find new environments and people nonthreatening and interesting. Animals are more likely to explore, test, and taste different food options presented during these critical periods of development. However, as this period of development passes, this window of "openness" closes. Animals become less receptive to new experiences, experimentation, and exploration. A mature animal may not recognize items with which it has had no prior experience as food. Such unfamiliarity can make it challenging to transition an adult animal to a healthier diet or allow for a wide variety of food options to be used to reinforce desired behavior. Exposing young parrots to a wide variety of foods, including different pellet types and fresh foods, can help prevent the challenges that often arise when transitioning parrots from seed-based diets. **Table 4** lists various strategies to help birds transition to healthier diets.

SUMMARY

Influencing animal behavior is an important part of companion animal care. Science-based training technology can be used to teach animals to cooperate in medical care, address behavior problems, and manage day-to-day interactions required for animal husbandry and care. Food can play a significant role in this process. Identifying preferred food and nonfood reinforcers, selectively reinforcing desired behaviors, and having an awareness of how food can influence behavior can help caregivers successfully manage the behavior of avian and exotic species.

SUPPLEMENTARY DATA

Supplementary data related to this article can be found online at http://dx.doi.org/10. 1016/j.cvex.2014.01.007.

REFERENCES

1. Chance P. First course in applied behavior analysis. Pacific Grove (CA): Brooks Cole Publishing Company; 1998. p. 462.
2. Heidenreich B. An introduction to the application of science based training technology. Vet Clin North Am Exot Anim Pract 2012;15:371–85.
3. Ramirez K. Husbandry. Animal training: successful animal management through positive reinforcement. Chicago: Shedd Aquarium Press; 1999. p. 549.
4. University of Southern Florida glossary for behavior analysis. Available at: http://www.coedu.usf.edu/abaglossary/main.asp. Accessed October 12, 2013.
5. Jensen GD. Preference for bar pressing over 'freeloading' as a function of number of rewarded presses. J Exp Psychol 1963;65:451–4.
6. Heidenreich BE. Managing the deliverance of food to create motivation. In: Proceedings Mid-Atlantic States Association of Avian Veterinarians. Mid-Atlantic States Association of Avian Veterinarians; 2006.
7. Edmonds M. Alternatives to the use of falconry equipment on nonraptors. In: Proceedings. International Association of Avian Trainers and Educators. International Association of Avian Trainers and Educators; 2002.
8. Heidenreich BE. Training birds for medical and husbandry behaviors. In: Proceedings Animal Behavior Management Alliance. Animal Behavior Management Alliance; 2004.
9. Heidenreich BE. The power of the secondary reinforcer. Expanding your list of reinforcers. In: Proceedings International Association of Avian Trainers. International Association of Avian Trainers; 2008.

10. Clark P. Diet linked behavior in parrots. Available at: http://www.pamela clarkonline.com/uploads/Diet-Linked_Behavior_in_Parrots.pdf. Accessed October 12, 2013.
11. Scott PS, Fuller JL. Genetics and social behavior of the dog. Chicago: The University of Chicago Press; 1965. p. 110–50.

Nutritional Support of Reptile Patients

Ryan S. De Voe, DVM, MSpVM, DACZM,
DABVP (Avian), DABVP (Reptile & Amphibian)

KEYWORDS

- Reptile • Nutrition • Assist feeding • Nutritional support • Neonates

KEY POINTS

- Nutritional support is a very important, though often neglected, factor in the management of sick and anorexic reptiles.
- Reptiles can benefit greatly from receiving appropriate nutritional support in a timely manner.
- A basic understanding of reptilian metabolism, digestive physiology, and the natural history of commonly encountered species can help the clinician make sensible recommendations for the maintenance of healthy animals and appropriate intervention in the case of ill animals.

INTRODUCTION

One of the most amazing characteristics of ectothermic animals is their gastrointestinal physiology and ability to efficiently process calories. Similarly sized mammals and reptiles use dramatically discordant amounts of calories and nutrients to function and grow. Though it is difficult to make broad statements regarding such huge and varied taxa, a generally accepted rule of thumb is that reptiles have approximately one-tenth of the energy requirements of a comparably sized mammal.[1,2] Because of the unique reptilian gastrointestinal physiology and energy metabolism, veterinarians are often confused about how to approach the nutritional support of ill reptiles. Many veterinarians and reptile keepers think that because reptiles in health do not eat as frequently as mammals or birds they can withstand the same kind of fasting intervals when clinically ill. Therefore, the tendency can be to allow ill reptiles to go considerable lengths of time before nutritional support is instituted. In many cases, short intervals of anorexia are not clinically important to the reptile but, in other cases, effective nutritional support can be the deciding factor as to whether or not treatment is successful.

North Carolina Zoological Park, 4401 Zoo Parkway, Asheboro, NC 27205, USA
E-mail address: ryan.devoe@nczoo.org

Vet Clin Exot Anim 17 (2014) 249–261
http://dx.doi.org/10.1016/j.cvex.2014.01.009
1094-9194/14/$ – see front matter © 2014 Elsevier Inc. All rights reserved.

Veterinarians will often recommend convalescing reptiles be kept at temperatures in the upper range of their preferred optimal temperature zone (POTZ) to increase their metabolic rate and speed healing.[3,4] The elevation in body temperature and metabolic rate associated with healing or recovery from illness increases the reptile patient's caloric needs independent of any other factors affecting the animal. Therefore, it is possible for reptile patients to develop a catabolic state when environmental temperatures are elevated and caloric intake does not address the increased needs.[5] This same issue can occur with healthy reptiles that are kept inappropriately warm without adequate caloric intake or which are not allowed to properly thermoregulate; however, the problem can become exacerbated with ill or injured animals.

Another important factor to consider in providing nutritional support is the effect digestion can have on metabolism in reptile patients. In several reptile species, researchers have documented what is referred to as specific dynamic action (SDA).[6] SDA is defined as an increase in metabolism caused by the ingestion of food, especially proteins, and is ubiquitous across a wide variety of animal taxa. In a study using pythons (Python regius and P molurus) ingestion of amino acids independent of body temperature resulted in a postprandial rise in oxygen consumption, heart rate, and growth of visceral organs,[7] which is representative of what has been seen in other vertebrate species. Thus, to maximize the metabolic rate and speed healing, reptiles should be given access to temperatures in the upper end of their POTZ and be fed adequately. Meal composition has an effect on SDA in reptiles, with meals having "complete" amino acid profiles (as found in whole vertebrate prey items) eliciting maximal effect compared with diets deficient in some amino acids. Fats and carbohydrates do not elicit SDA in reptiles.[8]

Though references exist regarding reptile nutrition, there is little solid research to guide the clinician when it comes to nutritional support of the reptile patient.[5] Therefore, much of what is presented in this article, though based on scientific fact, is anecdotal and it should be applied at the clinician's discretion according to details of the particular case.

Throughout this article, when referring to the feeding of whole prey items, it is assumed that the prey is prekilled unless otherwise specified.

CHOICE OF FOOD FOR ASSIST FEEDING

In most cases, unless there are specific contraindications, the animal's regular diet can be used for assist feeding. Many lizards and chelonians that are acclimated to people will readily accept hand feeding when they would otherwise refuse to eat. The author has seen several bearded dragons (Pogona vitticeps) and green iguanas (Iguana iguana) that become habituated to hand feeding and will refuse to eat food not presented by hand. Some anorexic reptiles (including snakes) will swallow a food item after it has been introduced into their mouths. One of the keys to success with this method in snakes is to hook the snake's teeth into the rodent so it is difficult for them to spit it out. This technique is described in further detail in the section on nutritional management of neonatal reptiles.

If the animal cannot or will not tolerate assist feeding with whole, natural food items, those food items can be liquefied in a blender or food processor and administered via gavage or an indwelling feeding tube. It may be necessary to dilute the resultant mixture so it will pass through an appropriately sized feeding tube. The author will often administer oral fluids as part of the treatment protocol, so the benefit of diluting food mixtures can be two-fold.

Currently, several commercially available products seem appropriate for providing nutritional support to reptile patients. Oxbow Animal Health (29012 Mill Rd, Murdoch NE, USA; www.oxbowanimalhealth.com) offers products formulated for herbivores (Herbivore Critical Care) and carnivores (Carnivore Critical Care). In addition, the Lafeber company (24981 N. 1400 East Rd, Cornell, IL, USA; www.lafeber.com) offers a variety of products with products formulated for herbivores and carnivores, as well as products created specifically for omnivores and piscivores. Anecdotally, these products have performed well in reptile patients. In some applications, these products offer an advantage over whole or natural food items because they are nutrient-dense, easily digested, and assimilated (ie, hydrolyzed proteins, amino acids). All of the afore-mentioned products come in a powdered form and they are reconstituted before administration. The author has occasionally experienced complications with the use of commercially available powdered diets. In these instances, following administration of the product, the material becomes dehydrated within the stomach or intestine and it creates an obstructive condition. This complication occurs when the patient is dehydrated and it can be avoided by paying careful attention to maintenance of adequate hydration. In most cases, resolution of this complication has been achieved by restoring normal systemic hydration and administration of oral fluids to rehydrate the food mass.

Historically many veterinarians have relied on canned "critical care" dog or cat diets for nutritional support of reptile patients. These foods are readily available and easy to use but may not be the best choice in most reptile cases and possibly detrimental in others. Critical care diets are formulated to contain highly digestible and calorically dense ingredients and many contain liver as primary ingredients. Liver is very high in purine content, which is a product of nucleotide degradation and precursor of uric acid.[9] In uricotelic reptiles, the ingestion of diets containing purine-rich ingredients will theoretically increase uric acid production and may exacerbate existing health conditions or create unnecessary complications. Clinicians should pay close attention to the ingredients of products they use to provide nutritional support to their reptile patients and make educated choices based on the physiology, age, and health of the particular species.

THE MECHANICS OF ASSIST FEEDING

Before administering nutritional support to a reptile patient, the animal must be properly conditioned to optimize benefit and avoid complications. First, the animal must be given access to an appropriate thermal gradient and allowed to thermoregulate. Some animals may not have normal mobility and, therefore, cannot behaviorally thermoregulate effectively. In these cases, the clinician will have to make a best guess on what temperature within the species POTZ the patient should be kept at. Regardless, with most reptile patients this means warming them up. If food is administered to an animal that has a body temperature less than what is necessary for digestion, putrefaction can occur within the gastrointestinal tract, creating a new array of problems to deal with. Following warming of the patient, the reptile needs to be adequately hydrated before feeding. If the animal is dehydrated, rehydration can be accomplished via administration of oral or parenteral fluids. Only after the animal has been brought to an appropriate body temperature and is considered normally hydrated should assist feeding be attempted.

As mentioned previously, many reptiles will accept assist feeding with minimal difficulty. When deciding on a method for providing nutritional support to a reptile patient, both human and reptile welfare must be considered. Working around the oral cavity of many reptiles puts the handler at serious risk of injury or even death with some venomous species (**Fig. 1**). Large chelonians and lizards, even if considered docile, can inflict severe wounds or even amputate digits should an accident occur during an assist-feeding episode. The animal can suffer as well if the handling necessary for the assist feeding is too rough or prolonged. The author's rule of thumb is that a reptile should not be vigorously restrained for more than 5 minutes at any one time, if possible. If assist feeding takes longer than 5 minutes and/or the animal fights the restraint unrelentingly, either chemical restraint or an indwelling feeding tube should be considered.

As previously stated, many reptiles can be assist fed simply by hand-offering food or placing food directly in the oral cavity. Syringe feeding a liquid diet is also possible when animals will tolerate it. Some lizards and chelonians will accept syringe feeding, though ultimately it depends on the individual patient's characteristics. When this is not possible, tube-feeding a liquid diet is often the next option. Tube feeding a reptile is similar to tube feeding avian patients and can be accomplished using either flexible or rigid tubes. Complications such as esophageal or gastric perforation can occur with either type of tube, so the type of tube should be based on clinician preference and patient characteristics. With a gentle touch, damage to the upper gastrointestinal tract due to tube feeding is rare. The author prefers tube feeding smaller reptiles with the stainless steel gavage tubes typically used with birds (**Fig. 2**). Red rubber catheters and larger rubber tubes can be used with larger patients. Care should be taken to ensure that the end of the tube is smooth and is passed gently to avoid trauma to the oral cavity, esophagus, and/or stomach. It is paramount that the animal be well restrained because even well-suited equipment used skillfully can cause damage to the animal if it breaks restraint. The judicious use of an appropriate oral speculum is

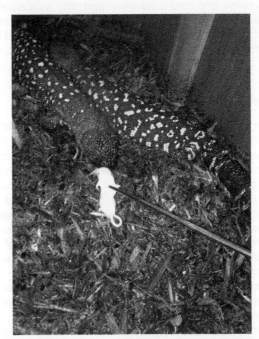

Fig. 1. Use of long hemostats for safe feeding of a venomous beaded lizard (*Heloderma horridum*).

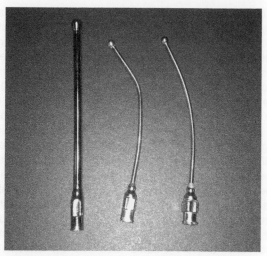

Fig. 2. Stainless steel feeding tubes used for gavage of small reptiles.

also recommended to avoid a variety of potential complications. If specula are not used, flexible tubes can be bitten off and swallowed and steel gavage tubes can induce injury to the oral or pharyngeal cavity and/or esophagus if an animal with sufficiently powerful jaws bites down on them. Oral specula also protect personnel performing the procedure from accidental bites.

When prolonged nutritional support is expected and/or the animal is difficult or dangerous to hand or tube feed, indwelling feeding tubes are indicated (**Fig. 3**). Placement of a pharyngostomy or esophagostomy tube is a simple surgical procedure within the realm of capability for most veterinary clinicians. With some reptiles, the act of assist feeding can be dangerous and stressful to both the animal and the human. Species that possess powerful jaws equipped with sharp teeth or beaks are formidable patients. Repeat administration of food or medications can be impractical,

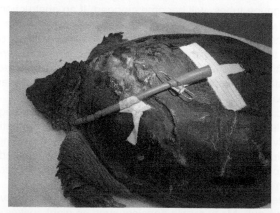

Fig. 3. An esophagostomy tube for long-term provision of nutritional support to a wild common snapping turtle (*Chelydra serpentina*) presented for rehabilitation. In this case, repeated feeding per os would be very stressful for the turtle and potentially dangerous for personnel.

stressful, unsafe, and ultimately counterproductive. Placement of a pharyngostomy or esophagostomy tube is indicated in any chronically anorexic patient that is not a serpent and that does not participate willingly in the assist-feeding process. Often, experienced reptile veterinarians will proactively place feeding tubes in anesthetized reptiles that they suspect may be unwilling to eat on recovery and during convalescence. In the author's practice, this is standard procedure with wild eastern box turtles (*Terapene carolina carolina*) that present for rehabilitation. Animals that are willing to eat voluntarily are rarely deterred by the presence of a feeding tube. Therefore, it is important that the animal continue to be given the opportunity to feed normally before every tube feeding. Once the animal is eating consistently, the tube can be removed and the defect will typically heal via second intention without complication.

Methods of tube placement are described elsewhere in detail, so will not be discussed in this paper. When placing the tube it is paramount to carefully verify its placement within the gastrointestinal tract. Usually this can be accomplished by pulling the tube out of the mouth and then redirecting down the esophagus, or direct visualization of the tube in place (using endoscopy if necessary). This step is critical to avoid the potential complication of delivering liquid food into the subcutaneous tissues or coelom of the patient. Another common mistake during pharyngostomy or esophagostomy tube placement is extension of the tube too far, resulting in perforation of the stomach or pressure necrosis of the gastric wall from the tube tip. The author typically administers a small amount of water-soluble contrast material such as diatrizoate via the feeding tube to verify proper placement before patient recovery from anesthesia. Though somewhat challenging in chelonian patients, proper tube placement can also be verified via ultrasonography. This method is made easier by flushing a small volume of saline through the tube to ideally create some distention of the stomach and confidence that the tip of the tube is appropriately positioned.

Maintenance of an indwelling feeding tube in reptiles can be challenging. The tube needs to be secured in a way that the animal will not easily dislodge it. Modification of the animal's environment to remove objects that the tube could be hung up on is also important. Before administration of food in to the feeding tube, it should be flushed with water to determine patency. It is also critical that the tube be aspirated before feeding to make sure the previously administered meal has left the stomach and is moving through the digestive tract appropriately. Occasionally, feeding tubes, especially very small gauge tubes, will become clogged. If an obstruction occurs, gentlly flushing the tube with warm water in a pulsatile fashion may be effective in restoring patency. Small amounts of dilute pineapple juice and/or vinegar can be routinely flushed through the tube with the idea that it will help breakdown concretions of food material within the tube. Feeding tubes can usually be replaced without too much difficulty after the tissues around the stoma have healed if an obstruction is intractable to clearance.

Indwelling feeding tubes are usually left in place until the reptile begins eating on its own. Most reptile patients will eat on their own when the condition causing the anorexia is resolved, despite the presence of the indwelling feeding tube. Follwing removal of the tube, the healed stoma can be surgically repaired; however, this does not seem to be necessary as closure of the stoma usually occurs rapidly with no intervention in otherwise healthy animals.

Deciding on the appropriate volume of food to deliver to a reptile via tube or assist feeding can be difficult. Many reptile species, such as giant snakes, monitor lizards, and crocodilians, are capable of ingesting huge meals relative to their body size. However, most reptile species are not capable of handling such large meals and should be fed conservatively. All cases need to be evaluated on an individual basis; however, a good starting point is 3% of bodyweight. This means that in the case of a 100 g animal, the initial volume of food to be delivered via tube feeding is 3 mL. This is not a perfect method because there is obviously variation in the weight of different liquid diets but it is close enough to provide a starting point. In most cases, the volume can be increased over time if desired. It should be understood this recommendation regarding volume of food administered is a general guideline and does not take into consideration nutrient density of the diet. Volume is typically the limiting factor when providing nutritional support to reptile patients, especially those that have been anorexic for some time. In starved avian patients that present to the author's wildlife rehabilitation center, the same rule of thumb for determining starting volume is used in combination with the calculated caloric requirements of the bird. In reptile patients, caloric requirements are not as well understood and vary depending on several factors. Therefore, the author has found providing nutritional support to reptiles based on volume to be an easier and more practical approach.

Gastrointestinal ileus is a common sequela of many conditions affecting reptile patients. For this reason, the clinician should carefully monitor patients for evidence of gastrointestinal dysfunction. When managing reptile cases that require nutritional support, the author will routinely mix barium sulfate into liquid diets or inject it in food items to easily track the food's transit through the gastrointestinal tract radiographically. This is a simple method to evaluate gastrointestinal motility and patency. Several publications report on the gastrointestinal transit time of various contrast materials in a variety of species. Transit times vary according to species and can range from approximately 1 to 7 days.[10–16]

REFEEDING SYNDROME

Otherwise healthy animals that experience physiologic anorexia (as seen during hibernation, torpor, or breeding) do not suffer from refeeding syndrome and they can be fed without concern even with considerable intervals between feedings. Some adult ball pythons (P regius) will only feed for 3 to 4 months out of the year but remain healthy, maintain body condition, and suffer no consequences when they begin to eat after months of anorexia. However, in animals that are ill, starved, and/or in a cachectic state, refeeding syndrome can result in significant morbidity.[5] Refeeding syndrome occurs when the acute influx of glucose causes life-threatening hypokalemia and hypophosphatemia. Development of refeeding syndrome can be avoided by conservative introduction of feeding following prolonged anorexic states. In these cases, it is best to correct any existing electrolyte abnormalities before feeding and limitation of initial food intake should not exceed 50% of what would be considered the animal's daily energy requirement.

NUTRITIONAL SUPPORT OF NEONATES

Neonatal reptiles can be tricky to manage nutritionally. Many reptiles are born or hatch with significant caloric stores via the internal yolk sac, which in the wild provides energy for dispersal before initiation of feeding. In the case of snakes, most species will go through ecdysis shortly after hatching or birth and do not typically feed until after this first shed. Usually this first ecdysis occurs within 10 to 14 days; however, some species, such as blood pythons (P curtus spp), do not shed for the first time until 3 to 5 months of age. Even with such prolonged intervals, these species do well clinically provided they are kept in a suitable habitat with ready access to water.

It is common to encounter neonatal reptiles suffering from acute hypoglycemia that will benefit greatly from nutritional support. Hatchling chelonians that have struggled to leave the egg and/or nest can present moribund but will respond dramatically to administration of a drop of oral 50% dextrose or other high-energy, easily absorbed food. The author has never measured blood glucose levels in neonatal reptiles that present in this condition (usually due to the diminutive size of the patient and benign nature of the intervention) but has seen many animals make surprising recoveries.

Another common dilemma with neonatal reptiles is some animals simply refuse to begin feeding following hatching or birth. Failure to begin feeding is most commonly encountered with snake species but it can occur with any taxa. Arboreal species and/or species that are especially diminutive as neonates are especially problematic. In the wild, these species typically take small frogs, lizards, or even invertebrates as their first prey, so that they do not recognize domestic neonatal mice as food is not surprising.

Several techniques are used by experienced herpetoculturists to entice anorexic neonatal snakes to feed. The reptile veterinarian should be aware of these techniques and implement them when possible. First, efforts should be made to create as suitable an environment as possible before offering the food item. The feeding attempt should be made during the time of day when the species is naturally most active and the environment should be calm and quiet. Another detail that is often overlooked is where the animal is fed. Many hobbyist publications recommend feeding reptiles outside of their enclosures to avoid habituating the animal to expect food every time the door to the cage opens. This is fine with well-established animals but completely disruptive to neonates that are not feeding consistently. In addition, arboreal species are much more likely to feed when on a comfortable perch. On the other end of the spectrum, fossorial species are more comfortable feeding when prey items are presented in covered areas such as under a piece of cork bark, sheet of newsprint, or in a hide box. In situations in which the prey item is being manipulated, a pair of long-handled forceps is recommended to maintain as much distance as possible between the keeper and animal, especially with venomous species. Many animals are not comfortable feeding in front of people and they will drop the prey item if they detect even the slightest movement in the environment, such as a withdrawing hand or someone walking away from the enclosure.

In cases in which an attempt is being made to feed rodent prey to a species that would normally begin feeding on amphibians or reptiles, manipulation of scent can be beneficial. Washing the rodent with a mild nonscented soap and rinsing thoroughly can help temper the odor of the rodent and improve palatability. Following washing, other scents can be applied to the rodent in an effort to make it smell like a frog, lizard, or other more natural prey. Scenting of rodents can be accomplished in a variety of ways. The simplest method is to take a lizard or frog and rub it on the rodent in an effort to transfer scent. Another method involves using a blender to make a frog or lizard slurry, which is applied to the food item. The author freezes opportunistically encountered road-killed frogs, toads, and lizards for this purpose. Live frogs and lizards can be used for scent transfer but their health and welfare should always be considered as part of the cost-benefit assessment. Pathogen transmission is possible with this practice but, if common sense is used and obviously diseased lizards or amphibians are avoided, the risk is often deemed acceptable.

Prekilled rodents can be manipulated to make them more attractive prey to neonatal snakes. If using frozen-thawed prey, care should be taken to ensure that the rodent is thoroughly thawed and is at a temperature similar to what would be considered normal for a rodent (around 100°F, 38°C). Often, detection of a warm object will elicit a strike and result in prehension and subsequent consumption of the prey item. Another useful trick is to incise the nose or head of the rodent to expose blood and tissue. This theoretically increases the presence of volatile material, which entices interest and a strike from the snake.

"Tease feeding" is another method that is used, especially with defensive arboreal species that will readily strike out and attempt to bite things that are disturbing them. Essentially, this practice involves eliciting a reflexive instinct that causes the snake to swallow the prey item once it is in their mouth. The prey item is held in a pair of forceps and used to annoy the snake until it strikes at, bites, and constricts or holds onto it. This procedure often requires multiple attempts and the key is holding still after the snake bites and holds onto the prey item. As previously mentioned, with some animals even slowly trying to back away can disturb the animal and redirect their attention causing them to drop the prey item.

If none of the aforementioned methods is successful, offering live rodents may be warranted. In the case of neonatal snakes, this usually means offering young pinkie mice and rats. Rodents this young present no danger compared with older rodents so there is no real downside to feeding live pinkies from the perspective of reptile health and safety. However, rodent welfare should not be ignored. The author considers the death of young rodents from hypothermia, dehydration, and/or starvation on the floor of an anorexic reptile's enclosure unacceptable.

Feeding neonatal snakes natural prey such as frogs, toads, and lizards is certainly a possibility if necessary or desired. It can be effectively argued this is a healthier and more natural approach to captive nutrition. The only reason rodents are preferred as food for captive snakes is availability and expense. Rodents are relatively cheap and plentiful. Though less available than rodents, "feeder" amphibians and lizards can be obtained through many dealers. In North America, invasive or common species are often collected and sold as feeder animals. Cuban tree frogs (Osteopilus sp), Mediterranean house geckos (Hemidactylus turcicus), and Anolis sp are frequently available. Feeder animals that are collected in the wild should be quarantined and screened properly to minimize the risk of disease transmission. Humane euthanasia and freezing for a period can help minimize, but does not completely negate, the risk of pathogen transmission.

In cases in which seemingly natural prey is offered, neonates may still stubbornly refuse to feed voluntarily. In these cases, experience suggests that it is best to begin assist feeding sooner rather than later. If assist feeding is delayed too long, many animals can become debilitated to the point at which intervention is futile. Various options exist for assist-feeding neonatal snakes. The first and easiest is the administration of a commercially available liquid diet. Whole prey items can be pureed and administered via the same method. Extruding devices, commonly referred to as a pinkie pumps, have been used for years by hobbyists to easily administer whole prey items to anorexic animals. Obviously, use of these tools necessitates humane euthanasia of the prey animal before administration. Another typically used method is assist feeding whole or large pieces of prey items. Adult mouse or rat tails are well suited for this purpose because of their shape. Obviously, rodent tails are not an appropriate long-term diet, but are suitable for the first few feedings if necessary. In these cases, the animal is well restrained and a lubricated food item is introduced into the oral cavity (**Fig. 4**). In some cases, the animal will instinctively swallow the prey from that point. The key to this procedure is hooking the teeth into the prey item so the snake cannot easily drop it. If the animal will not swallow the item voluntarily, it will need to be pushed down to the esophagus or stomach. This procedure should be approached with great care because it is easy to traumatize the reptile's upper gastrointestinal tract. In addition, some snakes will resist vigorously. If the procedure is not quickly completed, the negative effects of the stress the animal

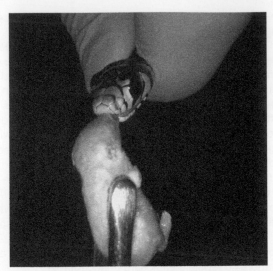

Fig. 4. Assist feeding a prekilled pinkie mouse to a young tiger ratsnake (*Spilotes pullatus*). The prey was introduced into the oral cavity and the snake was returned to its enclosure where it voluntarily swallowed the mouse.

experiences can outweigh the benefit of the feeding. If at any point during the feeding the animal noticeably weakens, the procedure should be aborted and future attempts should be modified to be less traumatic (eg, better restraint, smaller food item).

Some species of snakes are notoriously difficult to establish following birth or hatching. The author maintains a collection of pythons from the genus *Antaresia* (Children's, Stimson's, spotted, and pygmy pythons). These pythons make excellent captives because they are small, hardy, and often docile; however, the neonates can be challenging to work with. Patience and persistence will usually pay off but it can take many weeks to establish consistent voluntary feeding and, with clutches of 10 to 20 eggs, the commitment to succeed can be daunting. As an alternative, the author has found that, almost without fail, if neonatal *Antaresia* pythons are assist-fed a portion of a pinkie mouse following their first ecdysis, they will begin feeding voluntarily thereafter. Several other species respond similarly; therefore, if properly performed, this approach can be very effective. Not all species, or individual animals, will respond quickly to this technique. The author has worked with animals that have been anorexic for longer than a year following hatching or birth but eventually begin feeding vigorously on their own. Most memorably, a neonatal female green anaconda (*Eunectes murinus*) steadfastly refused food for almost 18 months. The snake was assist fed one to two appropriately sized mice or young rats every 7 to 10 days. Growth was reduced compared with voluntarily feeding littermates but it was appreciable. Before every assisted feeding, a rodent was presented with tongs to give the snake the opportunity to feed. One day the anaconda prehended and constricted the rodent enthusiastically and ever since it has fed voluntarily with gusto.

TIPS AND TRICKS FOR FEEDING CAPTIVE REPTILES
Monitors and Other Large, Carnivorous Lizards

Obesity with its associated complications is epidemic in captive monitor lizards. A monitor lizard in the wild is usually an extremely different beast from the sedentary, football-shaped lizards that are typically seen as pets. Wild monitors are typically lean, active hunters that feed opportunistically on almost anything they can run down and fit in their mouths. Captive monitors are typically fed diets consisting exclusively of laboratory rodents that are dangled right in front of their noses, whereas wild monitors consume a wide variety of food items that they have to work to capture. The natural diet of monitor species in the wild consists mostly of invertebrate prey but also includes eggs, fish, amphibians, and other reptiles. Mammals and birds are present in the natural diet but at very low levels.[17–19] The author has seen many obese monitor lizards with chronic colonic impactions consisting almost entirely of rodent hair. Not only does the colon become massively distended with feces, the development of transcolonic membranes will frequently concurrently occur.[20] Savannah monitors (*Varanus exanthematicus*) typically present with this disorder; therefore, when managing cases of constipation or obstipation in this species, colonic patency should always be verified early in the diagnostic investigation. Often, these cases are intractable to treatment by the time they are presented to a veterinarian. However, it is possible that these problems could be prevented with implementation of a more natural diet and increased exercise.

The author recommends as varied a diet as possible for captive varanid lizards, ideally consisting of at least 50% invertebrate prey. In addition, efforts should be made to encourage the animals to forage and expend energy. This can be accomplished with a variety of methods and keepers are encouraged to use their imagination. Minimally, if using prekilled rodents, chicks, or eggs, the prey items can be placed in various areas within the enclosure forcing the animal to forage. Invertebrate prey, such as crickets, mealworms, and cockroaches, are typically presented alive and require physical effort to capture them. Making the commitment to provide a diet such as this for a captive monitor lizard is difficult but rewarding because of the potential positive effects for the animal.

GRASSLAND TORTOISES

It is important to recognize that not all tortoise species require the same diet. A common mistake is to offer diets that are too rich to grassland species such as leopard (*Geochelone pardalis*) and sulcata (*G sulcata*) tortoises. These tortoises will greedily consume large amounts of fruit and vegetables (not to mention animal protein and waste, if given the opportunity); however, in the wild they rarely encounter such food items and eat most low-quality grasses and vegetation. A grassland tortoise on an appropriate diet consisting of more than 90% grass will have formed, relatively dry, droppings, which are composed mostly of compressed stems. Compare this to a tortoise that receives large amounts of chopped fruits, vegetables, and leafy greens, which will have loose and smelly droppings.

Grassland tortoises will usually feed daily in the wild but in captivity many are offered food only a few times a week. Much like small herbivores such as rabbits and rodents, constant grazing is beneficial for the gastrointestinal function and health of grassland tortoises. A healthy well-fed sulcata tortoise will have ingesta and feces in the entirety of its gastrointestinal tract at all times.

Many well-intentioned keepers will offer grass hays to their captive tortoises directly from the bale. The choice of food is correct but the method of presentation can cause problems. When offered cut hay, tortoises often ingest entire (indigestible) stems intact. These stems can accumulate and result in gastrointestinal impactions, especially in smaller animals. When grazing naturally, tortoises will tear the stems as they pull a mouthful away from the rooted plant, creating a much shorter and more manageable strand length. A simple way to avoid problems with stem length is to chop the hay before offering it to the tortoise. A good rule of thumb is not to feed stems longer than the length of the tortoises' plastron.

FEEDING FREQUENCY

Most captive reptiles are not fed on a daily basis. As previously discussed, the theory behind this feeding strategy is that, as ectotherms, reptiles do not require daily caloric intake and their relatively infrequent feeding is healthy or at least not detrimental. With the exception of some snakes, crocodilians, and lizards that binge and ingest prey items that are gigantic relative to their body size, most reptiles will eat daily during their active times of the year if possible. In animals that naturally eat more frequently, the down-regulation of gastrointestinal function is much less dramatic between meals compared with "binge" eaters.[21] Therefore, these animals commit relatively more caloric resources toward maintenance of their gastrointestinal tracts in between meals. As a result, insectivorous and small omnivorous or herbivorous lizards and turtles do well when fed daily. Even giant snakes do well in captivity when fed smaller frequent meals versus occasional large meals. It is the author's impression that snakes fed in this manner are more active and maintain better body condition compared with those fed large prey infrequently. It is possible to create overweight animals regardless of feeding frequency, thus growth and/or body condition must be continually monitored and the amount of food offered per feeding adjusted accordingly.

SUMMARY

Nutritional support is an important, though often neglected, factor in the management of sick and anorexic reptiles. Reptiles can greatly benefit from receiving appropriate nutritional support in a timely manner. A basic understanding of reptilian metabolism, digestive physiology, and the natural history of commonly encountered species can help the clinician make sensible recommendations for the maintenance of healthy animals and appropriate intervention in the case of ill animals.

REFERENCES

1. Bennet AF, Dawson WR. Metabolism. In: Gans C, Dawson WR, editors. Biology of the reptilian. Physiology A, vol. 5. London: Academic Press; 1976. p. 127–211.
2. Karasov WH, Diamond JM. Digestive adaptations for fueling the cost of endothermy. Science 1985;228(4696):202–4.
3. O'Malley B. General anatomy and physiology of reptiles. In: Clinical anatomy and physiology of exotic species. Edinburgh (Ireland): Elsevier Saunders; 2005. p. 17–40.
4. Mitchell M. Therapeutics. In: Mader DR, editor. Reptile medicine and surgery. St Louis (MO): Saunders; 2006. p. 631–64.
5. Donoghue S. Nutrition. In: Mader DR, editor. Reptile medicine and surgery. St Louis (MO): Saunders; 2006. p. 251–98.
6. Wang T, Busk M, Overgaard J. The respiratory consequences of feeding in amphibians and reptiles. Comp Biochem Physiol A Mol Integr Physiol 2001;128(3):535–49.
7. Enok S, Simonsen LS, Wang T. The contribution of gastric digestion and ingestion of amino acids on the postprandial rise in oxygen consumption, heart rate and growth of visceral organs in pythons. Comp Biochem Physiol A Mol Integr Physiol 2013;165(1):46–53.

8. BiMcCue MD, Bennett AF, Hicks JW. The effect of meal composition on specific dynamic action in Burmese pythons (*Python molurus*). Physiol Biochem Zool 2005;78(2):182–92.

9. Mader DR. Gout. In: Mader DR, editor. Reptile medicine and surgery. St Louis (MO): Saunders; 2006. p. 793–800.

10. Hatch KA, Aflick D. Retention time of digesta in insectivorous lizards—a comparison of methods and species. Comp Biochem Physiol A Mol Integr Physiol 1992; 124(1):89–92.

11. Smith D, Dobson H, Spence E. Gastrointestinal studies in the green iguana: technique and reference values. Vet Radiol Ultrasound 2001;42(6):515–20.

12. Taylor SK, Citino SB, Zdiarski JM, et al. Radiographic anatomy and barium sulfate transit time of the gastrointestinal tract of the leopard tortoise (*Testudo pardalis*). J Zoo Wildl Med 1996;27(2):180–6.

13. Long CT, Page RB, Howard AM, et al. Comparison of Gastrografin to barium sulfate as a gastrointestinal contrast agent in red-eared sliders (*Trachemys scripta elegans*). Vet Radiol Ultrasound 2010;51(1):42–7.

14. Santos AQ, Lopes LR, Ferreira CG, et al. Determination of gastrointestinal transit in *Podocnemis expansa*. PUBVET 2011;5(12). No pagination.

15. Banzato T, Russo E, Finolti L, et al. Development of a technique for contrast radiographic examination of the gastrointestinal tract in ball pythons. Am J Vet Res 2012;73(7):996–1001.

16. Valiente AL, Marco I, Parga ML, et al. Ingesta passage and gastric emptying times in loggerhead sea turtles (*Caretta caretta*). Res Vet Sci 2008;84(1):132–9.

17. Bennett D. Diet of juvenile *Varanus niloticus* (Sauria: Varanidae) on the Black Volta River in Ghana. J Herpetol 2002;36(1):116–7.

18. Fiorenzo G. Diet of a large carnivorous lizard, *Varanus varius*. Wildl Res 2001; 28(6):627–30.

19. Sutherland DR. Dietary niche overlap and size partitioning in sympatric varanid lizards. Herpetologica 2011;67(2):146–53.

20. Chinnadurai SK, De Voe RS. Diagnosis, management and possible etiology of a transcolonic membrane in a savannah monitor (*Varanus exanthematicus*). J Herp Med Surg 2008;18(3/4):123–6.

21. Christel CM, DeNardo DF, Secor SM. Metabolic and digestive response to food ingestion in a binge-feeding lizard, the Gila monster (*Heloderma suspectum*). J Exp Biol 2007;210(19):3430–9.

Considerations and Conditions Involving Protozoal Inhabitation of the Reptilian Gastrointestinal Tract

Adolf K. Maas III, DVM, DABVP (Reptile and Amphibian Practice)

KEYWORDS

- Gastroenteritis • Parasites • Reptile • Chelonia • Protozoan • Virulence
- Superinfection • Squamate

KEY POINTS

- Gastrointestinal protozoal inhabitation does not equate with parasitism.
- Superinfections increase the virulence of protozoan infestations.
- Identification of the protozoan(s) present is essential to the treatment plan.
- Systemic health must be considered when determining treatment options

PARASITISM

Parasitism is any situation at which one set of DNA is replicated with the help of—and at the expense of—another set of DNA.[1]

A parasite is, in its simplest definition, an organism that lives at the expense of another individual, the host. In modern definition the parasite is a eukaryote, thus removing all bacteria and viruses from this category. It may be protozoan or metazoan, protist, fungal, plant or animal, and may have the ability to infect a host from the same or a completely different phylogenetic kingdom. A parasite may have a single host or multiple hosts, or may require a series of different hosts while it completes its life cycle. The greatest commonality between parasites is that they place an expense on the life cycle of their host. Also relevant is the medical aspect that a parasite is also an organism that needs to be removed for the sake of the health of the host.

The counterpoint to a parasitic relationship is that of a symbiotic relationship. Symbiosis is defined as a situation whereby both organisms receive mutual net benefit from their association. The best example might be that of zooxanthellae algae inhabiting cnidarian endoderm, where the intracellular algae provides a food source from photosynthesis to the coral or anemone while the host cnidarian provides protection

ZooVet Consulting, PLLC, PO Box 1007, Bothell, WA 98041, USA
E-mail address: drmaas@zoovet.us

Vet Clin Exot Anim 17 (2014) 263–297
http://dx.doi.org/10.1016/j.cvex.2014.01.008
1094-9194/14/$ – see front matter © 2014 Elsevier Inc. All rights reserved.

and nutrition for the algae. Neither of these organisms are able to survive well, nor for very long, without continuing their intimate association. By contrast, in a parasite/host relationship the parasite cannot survive without its host(s), whereas the host will continue its life cycle without the parasite. However, true symbiotic relationships are rare in comparison with parasitism.

A further definition for a parasite is that of "an organism that grows, feeds and/or is sheltered on or in a separate organism, while contributing nothing to the survival of that organism." Although this is more elegantly defined, the error lies in that this definition overlaps with that of a commensal relationship, whereby one organism lives in close association with another organism in such a way that one species benefits without harm to the other. There is debate as to whether true commensalism exists; in nearly all cases examined there is benefit to the organism while there is a small, but measurable detriment to the host. Thus, commensalism is subjective, as whether or not a host/parasite relationship is commensal is determined based on whether the analyst assesses the loss to the host as "significant".

The definition of "expense" to the host is the underlying issue in these terms. Many things can influence the definition of the expense to the host, and these influences themselves can be variable depending on what other factors are influencing the overall condition of the host. Just as bacteria inhabiting an organism can play different roles, so can eukaryotic and metazoan organisms vary their effect on their host.

Thus, rather than strict definitions, there is a continuum of these associations between a host and a presumptive parasite (or commensal, or symbiont) (**Fig. 1**).

Theoretically, a truly commensal or symbiotic organism would be placed at the left end of the continuum shown, whereas a true, aggressive parasite would be placed to the right. In reality, no organism could survive if it was truly located at either extreme. A parasite that caused an acutely lethal condition in its host would not be able to persist and survive to future generations, whereas a "parasite" that gained nothing and had no effect on its host would also not likely survive because it would be expending more energy to maintain its relationship than it would gain (however, under this definition the host and parasite roles might be reversed). To compound matters further, where then should the organism be placed that, under certain conditions, might have no negative effect on the host, but where under different conditions is detrimental to the health of the host?

The problems then lie in determining the effect the purported parasite has on its host, and thus assessing an organism as a parasite. It is simple to apprehend that an organism that reduces the energy, or causes a systemic disease, or prevents the host from reproducing can be defined as a parasite, but how should the ones that cause negligible or poorly defined issues truly be construed as a parasite requiring treatment? The solution might lie in asking the following questions:

1. Does the "parasite" affect the energy balance of the host?
2. Does the "parasite" affect the host's immune system (stimulatory or inhibitory)?

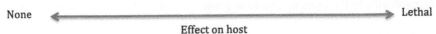

None ←――――――――――――――――――――――――――――――→ Lethal

Effect on host

Fig. 1. A continuum of associations between a host and a presumptive parasite (or commensal, or symbiont). Please note that the consideration of a positive effect on the host is not considered here, because to be accurate this would have to be a second axis intersecting the line above. There is supportive evidence that known parasites can provide a benefit to the host, in addition to the benefits that occur from symbiotic relationships, and that negative effects are "mathematically" erased by the presence of positive effects.

3. Is the host affected in other (nonenergy, nonimmunomodulating) ways, perhaps in other systems?
4. Does the infected host have deviations in behaviors from noninfected individuals?
5. Is there physical damage caused to the host by the "parasite"?

In theory, if the answer to any of these questions is yes, the organism should be deemed a parasite and treatment is required. Following this logic, however, any mammalian embryo produced during gestation is, without question, also a parasite, requiring treatment. Therefore, further evaluation to determine the pathologic effect of any purported parasite needs to be considered.

WHAT IS A CLINICAL PARASITE?

A clinical parasite is, simply stated, any parasitic organism inhabiting a host organism that is causing detriment to the host to the point that clinical intervention is advised. Unfortunately this is a subjective concept, one that requires not only knowledge of the parasite involved but also the effects on the host and evaluation of the significance of those effects. In all instances of parasites, the most important thing to consider is that they cannot survive without their host(s), whereas their host can survive without them. Granted, it is likely that this may be the case in symbiotic relationships as well, but because neither symbiont would survive if the other were not present, one could also state that each species was playing the role of the parasite.

Furthermore, the veterinarian also requires knowledge of the intervention options (therapeutic), the alternative (side) effects of the therapy, and an assumption as to the outcome of the therapy. First, however, a "typical" parasite must be examined.

Traditionally when one considers a readily identifiable parasite, a tapeworm easily comes to mind. The tapeworm is the classic metazoan parasite, one that most, if not all, people conjure invoke the term is presented. The classic evolutionary definition of a parasite is adhered to, in that tapeworms are organisms that have replaced portions of their anatomy and physiology with that of the function and structure of their host in the adaptation to remove systems no longer necessary for their success. In the case of a tapeworm, there is a very simple animal that has no eyes, no mouth, no intestine (with the beautiful simplicity of having its "intestinal" digestive and absorptive structures on the outside of its body[2]), having only retained the organizing center (analogous to a brain), a remarkable endocrine/exocrine system, the structures to attach itself within its host, the ability to be motile, and reproductive organs (albeit hermaphroditic, no longer necessitating a second individual to reproduce): in short, an organism at its simplest.

In and of the adaptations that it has taken on, a tapeworm is an organism that also cannot survive without its host(s). Granted, the specificity of a parasite to a host (ie, a parasite may require only a single specific host, such as *Eimeria caviai*, or may have a wide range of hosts, such as *Toxoplasma gondii*) may be variable, but every parasite depends on its host(s) to survive. The adaptations that a tapeworm's ancestors developed, while optimizing them to a specific environment (the host), have eliminated the possibility of pursuing alternative lifestyles. It is easy to say, then, that parasites have discarded portions of themselves as a complete organism in an effort to follow Darwinian law and best adapt themselves for success in their environment.

The clinical importance of a parasite is the measureable effect on its host. The hallmarks for tapeworm infections are vitamin B deficiencies, weight loss, and alterations in gastrointestinal motility. The parasites absorb nutrients from the host's digestive tract and grow, sometimes to the point that the host cannot obtain sufficient nutrition and will then lose body condition. Physical changes are also identified with tapeworm infestations; intestinal mucosal and submucosal lesions where the parasites are or have been attached, and systemic inflammatory changes, are commonly identified.[3] Motility changes in the host gut are seen with chronic infections, and there are indications that tapeworms, like many parasites, secrete compounds that significantly influence host gastrointestinal function.[4,5]

Granted, the full scope of a tapeworm infestation is not considered here. Only superficial primary host effects are reviewed; intermediate-stage infections, paratenic infections, and infections into accidental or dead-end hosts are not brought into consideration. Furthermore, there can be profound multiple systemic effects in any host with these infestations.[6–8] These effects are not reviewed here, as this is only a brief evaluation of whether a tapeworm should be considered as a clinical parasite.

It must be remembered that the effects seen on the host in most parasitic relationships are rarely as well defined as they are in the case of tapeworms. These effects are often multisystemic, and may not even be casually observable. However, in all cases the effect (or known potential effect) on the host is what determines if treatment is indicated. The evaluation of these effects on an entire population is the assessment of pathogenicity.

PATHOGENICITY AND VIRULENCE

In the practice of medicine there is a constant evaluation of any condition as to whether to treat. In infectious conditions, this determination relies on the pathogenicity of the infecting organism and the ability to exert damage on its host. As would be expected, commensal organisms are not thought to have the capacity to damage their host under this definition. However, this is not always the case, and more data are being produced demonstrating that commensal organisms may have the ability to cause pathologic conditions and that identified parasites do not always damage their host.[9]

As pathogenicity is considered an innate function of a pathogenic organism to damage a host organism, commensal and opportunist organisms, by definition, lack this inherent ability. However, parasites can express a wide range of disorder on their host organisms, and disease is not a guaranteed outcome of infection. Virulence, however, refers to the degree of pathologic status caused by an organism. The extent of this disorder may be affected by both intrinsic and extrinsic factors from both the parasite and the host, and can vary between individuals. Thus, virulence is a more relevant term for parasites, as parasitism has been found to be associated with nonpathogenic cases whereas commensals may cause abnormality. Under this term, virulence may be applied to all host-parasite relationships, eliminating the need for the term commensal, with any parasite then having an assessment of its virulence.

Therefore, determination of an organism's virulence to the individual host is key to the determination of whether said infection requires treatment. Note that whereas this may be a general call for treatment with some parasites in which a high innate virulence has been established, it also requires case-specific evaluation in instances where the virulence is low, unknown, or poorly established.

One measure of whether to treat should also be the level of virulence and pathology seen with endemic infections in wild populations of the host species. If the endemic virulence is high, treatment is likely indicated, as this suggests that the virulence is a genetic factor of the parasite. However, low endemic virulence does not mean that treatment is not required, as infestations of captive reptiles may have a variable level of virulence. This variability can be due to extrinsic factors found in captivity. Examples of such factors include superinfections, stress, and coinfections.

Superinfections

Superinfections denote that a host is repeatedly infected with either the same species or other species of parasite without the ability to naturally reduce or clear the parasite load between infections. In captive populations, reptiles are typically housed in a small enclosure (in comparison with wild animal ranges). As these animals often defecate within their cage and in their water source, they contaminate their environment. Furthermore, sanitation will almost always be substandard when compared with a wild animal's home range, which usually has rain and sunlight (ultraviolet) to sanitize the soil, moving water to remove infective agents (oocysts, ova, and so forth), and a great deal of area to contaminate with fecal material, often not encountered again by the same individual. Thus, because of their environment captive animals will continually be reexposed to a source of infection, creating a higher infection load than normally seen in wild individuals and not allowing for normal reduction of the parasite load.

Superinfections have also been found to develop a higher virulence than a regular infection, likely because of the increased number of parasitic organisms present and the increased competition seen between the parasites (**Fig. 2**).[10] Thus superinfections, when identified, strongly suggest a need for treatment.[11]

Stress

All animals, in all conditions, undergo stress. Stress in wild reptiles may include predation, food competition, reproductive performance, and other factors. However, captivity presents stress factors not otherwise seen in wild populations. Inappropriate husbandry, such as incorrect temperature levels, inadequate ultraviolet light, inappropriate light cycles, poor diet, and lack of proper enclosure enrichment are some of the most common stressors found to affect a captive reptile. Other forms of stress, such as forced contact with conspecifics within (and within visible range of) the enclosure and environmental peripheral activities (dogs barking, handling, television images, peripheral odors/chemicals, and so forth) seem to be more commonly disregarded but likely still have a role in the general health of the animal. Any stressor has the potential to make the host animal more susceptible to disease, and thus can have an effect on the virulence of the parasite.

Coinfections

Concurrent infections with pathogenic bacteria or viruses have a profound effect on any animal's immune system, and it can be easily discerned how a coinfection of one or more of these could allow a low-virulence parasitic infection to cause more serious disease. There are reports of coinfections in reptiles and discussions of the pathologic conditions observed.[12,13]

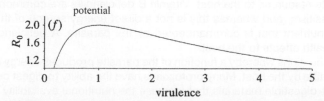

Fig. 2. The equilibrium distribution of parasitic strains with different virulences. The x-axis denotes virulence and the y-axis indicates frequencies. (*From* Nowak MA, May RM. Superinfection and the evolution of parasitic virulence. Proc R Soc Lond B 1994;255:83; with permission. Copyright © 1994, The Royal Society.)

Establishing the source of the parasite may assist in determining the virulence. Simply the presence of a parasite or infectious agent within a reptile does not constitute an infection. Many families of reptiles are strict carnivores/insectivores, with still more groups being omnivorous. Pseudoparasites, specifically rodent pinworms, mammalian mites, and cricket eggs, have been documented in the feces of reptiles that have eaten mammals or crickets. Insect-eating insects have been found to possess gastrointestinal protozoa that they do not normally harbor until they have ingested them via infected prey.[14] A study evaluating coccidian parasites in a wild population of house geckoes (*Hemidactylus frenatus*) found a known protozoal parasite of invertebrates within fecal samples.[15] This coccidian specie's natural history is known not to include vertebrates, so the conclusion was that the presence of the oocysts was as a pseudoparasite. No studies have been completed, but there is speculation that insect gut flora may be being detected in fecal samples of captive reptiles and is being overinterpreted as a parasitic infection. Therefore, the observation of protozoa in a gastrointestinal tract sample from a prey-consuming reptile does not automatically constitute a case of parasitism but rather indicates a need for further investigation.

ASSESSING THE NEED FOR TREATMENT

How can the need for treatment be assessed, particularly in those cases of gastrointestinal parasites where the effects may be occult? Unfortunately, there are few specific markers that can be objectively evaluated to assess virulence, the effect of a parasite on its host. As "necropsy is the ultimate diagnosis" (H. Steinberg, DVM, PhD, DACVP, personal communication, 2000), the virulence can then be accurately assessed using this technique, although this is not a particularly attractive means when survivability of the individual host animal is a concern. Thus, other methods should be considered for such determination.

If one returns to the questions posed earlier, the answers may be helpful in determining whether treatment is advised.

Does the Parasite Disrupt the Energy/Nutritional Balance of the Host?

This assessment relates to the net drain the parasite places on its host, not whether the parasite uses resources belonging to the host. The most obvious determination is whether the parasite uses metabolic energy otherwise needed by the host. With gastrointestinal parasites, there may be an excess of utilizable energy in the intestines (or cecum, or stomach, or cloaca) that the purported parasite is using for its own purposes. Thus with low-level infestations there may not be any net loss of available energy to the host. However, with significant infections, the parasite load may take up a large amount of available energy and the host may be in an energy deficit.

Coupled with this is the question as to whether the parasite reduces the amount of other available resources to the host. Vitamin B deficiencies are common with many types of parasitism, and whereas this is not a direct energy source of the host, it is an essential nutrient that is commandeered by the parasite. A deficiency will have significant health effects to the host.

There are situations whereby a function of the parasite produces energy or products that are utilizable by the host. Many protozoans have the ability to digest cellulose and produce host-digestible materials that increase the nutritional availability of the food they ingest. Tortoises and iguanas often have intestinal and cecal inhabitants (both protozoan and metazoan) that have the capacity to assist in the breakdown of the herbaceous material, which the host does not have endogenously. As there is likely more product than what is required by the flora, nutrition is increased to the host animal.

Thus, whereas the "parasites" may consume metabolic materials and deny the host the ability to access them, they also contribute other metabolic products that measure out at a net zero balance, or better. Again, positive and negative effects do not automatically cancel each other out, so although food increases and consumption may result in a zero change, an increase in energy availability and a vitamin B deficiency do not offset each other.

Does the Parasite Affect the Host's Immune System?

Inflammation in infected systems is a hallmark of any infection/infestation. It is not uncommon to identify a systemic inflammatory response in reptilian gastroenteritis.[16] However, many parasites do not appear to cause significant systemic inflammation in low-grade infestations.

Stress, as discussed earlier, can be exacerbated by a parasitic infestation just as easily, as parasitic infections can be worsened by external sources of stress. In intestinal parasitism there is the potential for ulcerations, abscesses, diverticuli, and blockages to occur, in addition to nutritional dyscrasias. All of these changes may cause stress. In all animals studied, stress causes increases of catabolic steroids such as cortisol and analogues, which have been well demonstrated to decrease inflammatory responses, increase healing times, and suppress many symptoms associated with disease. Thus, stress caused by disease associated with parasitism will have an effect on the host's immune system.

Is the Host Affected in Other (Nonenergy, Nonimmunomodulating) Ways, Perhaps in Other Systems?

This aspect can often be difficult to assess in the typical case of gastrointestinal parasitism, but the indirect signs are often readily seen. There are many reports of anorexia, diarrhea, and other associated conditions. Fluid balance can be affected as easily as the energy balance, and although reptiles typically can handle wide deviations in electrolyte levels with no effect, variations outside of their safe physiologic ranges can persist with little symptomology until the condition of the animal is so weak that it can no longer suppress it. Even neurologic signs can be seen with parasitism, but it may be difficult to discern whether they are primary or secondary. Some reptilian parasites may have multisystemic effects and can infect many other systems besides the gastrointestinal tract, or may infect the gastrointestinal tract in addition to the other sites.

Does the Host Have Deviations in Behaviors from Noninfected Individuals?

Behavior changes of the host caused by its parasites are well documented in a wide variety of parasites as well as their effect on their host in everything from insects[17] to rodents.[18] This assessment may be considered more difficult in reptiles, as the study of these animals' behavior both in their natural environment and in captivity is still in its infancy. However, changes in behaviors are often the impetus on owners or caretakers have lead them to bring reptiles to the clinic for examination and treatment. These changes are often relatively minor, such as increased basking/heat-seeking, activity change, or changes in appetite such as increased, decreased, or selective feeding.

Is There Physical Damage Caused to the Host by the "Parasite"?

External parasites and intermediate-stage parasites (ie, sparganosis and so forth) can easily be seen to cause physical damage to the host, but damage is often difficult to assess in the reptile patient with gastrointestinal protozoal parasitism. As stated earlier, physical changes can occur in the gastrointestinal tract as a direct result of the infestation, but some specific parasites have been found to infect multiple systems[19] with the gastrointestinal tract possibly not the primary site of damage. Some primary intestinal parasites have been identified and are pathogenic within other systems.[20]

Additional Considerations

Ancillary testing can also play a role in the determination of virulence and, thus, a need for treatment. Serum chemistries may show indication of tissue damage (focusing on the possibility of gastrointestinal damage) but interpretation can be difficult, as there are few specific markers and wide variations between species. This variation can be compounded with a paucity of established reference ranges in many genera. Serum electrophoresis (EPH) may be helpful as a means to assess inflammatory response, but conclusions will be limited because interpretation of EPH results is still considered to be in its infancy within herpetologic medicine. A complete blood count of the host may or may not indicate an active inflammatory process, anemia, or other secondary response of the host to infestation. However, there is no single test that will allow for a complete assessment of virulence, and any combination of these, plus many others, should be used in addition to clinical presentation in attempting to ascertain virulence in a patient.

Although diagnostic testing for the identification of specific parasites is discussed in more detail later in this article, the central goal is to discern between a primary pathogenic infection, an intermediate parasite with variable virulence, and a commensal organism whose only offense is of presence.

The dietary nature of the reptile should be considered when diagnosing parasitism. Carnivores are common hosts for many gastrointestinal parasites. Their prey often is the intermediate host (ie, *Sarcocystis*), or they may be asymptomatic carriers for parasitic organisms that are virulent after ingestion by a carnivore (ie, *Cryptosporidium*). Thus, assessing the specific diet of the host is necessary to determine risk and potential virulence, as well as the cause of the disease.

Insectivores create a more difficult paradigm to determining parasitism. Not only do the same concerns as with carnivorous reptiles arise, but many insects (particularly prey species used for captive reptiles) also contain protozoal organisms and parasites within their system. These protozoans are generally not known to cause abnormality in reptiles, but are commonly passing through the gut of the predatory reptile after ingesting the host insect. This process creates the problem of determining whether the protozoa observed in a fecal sample is a type that is related to the symptoms (in ill reptiles), has the potential for virulence (in asymptomatic reptiles), or is merely a pseudoparasite.

Herbivorous reptiles have still different issues in determination of whether a protozoal species may have virulence in its host. As it is unlikely that herbivores will ingest protozoa inhabiting their food items that will remain alive through their gastrointestinal tract (with the exception of cysts), this is less of a concern. However, all herbivores practice some form of fermentative digestion using protozoal and bacterial systems to assist in the breakdown of their ingesta. The residential flora may likely be superficially similar in appearance to parasitic organisms. Therefore, a thorough knowledge of normal protozoan and metazoan flora is necessary to assess potential virulence.

As a concept in assessing virulence, the benefits obtained by the host from the parasite need to be considered. As already mentioned, there is the obvious: protists may have a significant role in the conversion of indigestible plant fiber into a usable food source for the host that provides it with raw materials and a constant environment to live in. Returning to the concept of a tapeworm as a parasite, the detriments to an infection are well documented, but recently possible immunologic benefits have been identified, with chronic, low-grade infestations having a role in relieving chronic gastrointestinal inflammation and diarrhea.[21] In addition, the modification of prey (intermediate host) by a parasite to make it more easily captured by the predator is also demonstrated in many cases. Of note, studies have shown that parasites that use trophic transmission in the intermediate hosts generally have low virulence in the definitive host.[22] Furthermore, there are many studies in the human literature showing some correlation between asymptomatic parasite loads and improved health, such as a decreased incidence in allergies in children. These health improvements have not yet been completely proved or well understood, but if the correlations become causations, this would become a strong argument for the coevolution of any organism with the parasites that inhabit it.

Even though all reptiles may have normal protozoal flora, there is still the concern of increased virulence as a result of increased competition in cases of populations in excess of normal.[11] In many cases of parasitism in reptiles this is a difficult assessment, whether because of inexperience of the clinician reviewing the samples or because there are insufficient data regarding normal levels, or simply because there is no known assessment for the particular species. Ruminant medicine is an excellent example from which to draw knowledge. The determination of parasitic virulence is assessed not simply by the presence of an organism, but rather the density of the organism in a fecal sample. *Giardia* are considered to be normal flora within the gastrointestinal tract of chinchillas (*Chinchilla lanigera*), but are assessed to be at a pathogenic level when they are present in numbers above a threshold population.[23] Although the determination of parasite counts and threshold levels have not been completed for any herpetologic species, this concept should still be applied so as not to eliminate organisms that may provide a benefit to the host. Put simply, this means that every case of possible gastrointestinal parasitism needs to be evaluated individually to include the natural history of the host, stressors in the host's environment, and a review of what is currently known regarding acceptable parasite loads for that species.

Biological economics are a factor in parasite virulence. High exploitation rates may produce high fecundity and potentially increased transmission rates, but may also limit the amount of time the host will be able to provide resources. In addition, there has been evidence that pathogens adopt decreased virulence levels as they become more host adapted. Through lower exploitation rates, the parasite can inhabit a single host for potentially a significantly longer time, have a higher net reproduction rate, and increase the possible exposure rate to other potential hosts.[24] The process of host adaptation is only as rapid as the generation time of the pathogen; organisms that have the fastest generational times adapt to their host the quickest. Protists are continually adapting to best survive in their environment, and they have relatively short generational time. This fact may explain why so many virulent protist parasites resemble their nonvirulent or low-virulent relatives. The organisms with low virulence may have established because they caused little to no morbidity and so were better suited to surviving in their host without conflict with the host's immune system.

Lastly, has Koch's Postulate been satisfied? Koch's Postulate is considered to be the determinant factor in deciding whether or not an organism is a pathogen. However, few studies have been done to assess most purported parasites in reptiles. Protozoa that were originally assessed to be nonpathogenic are now understood to have variable virulence. It is clear that more studies need to be undertaken with methods that will help us understand the host-parasite relationship, assess virulence, and determine a methodology that will provide an evidence-based treatment plan when needed.

ZOONOSES

The consideration of zoonotic risks should also be a factor when considering treatment of a parasite infestation. Although reptiles are intermediate or paratenic hosts for many types of helminths, there are few data to suggest that protozoal parasites may be zoonotic from reptiles. However, despite there being no conclusion that protozoan parasites are zoonotic, there is also no indication that they are also not zoonotic (Eric Klaphake, DVM, DACZM, DABVP, personal communication, 2013).

An increasing body of data is demonstrating that *Cryptosporidium* species that were originally thought to be singular are in fact clades and very host specific.[25] Further division of these species is warranted for a complete understanding of their life cycles.[26] Until these species are studied in depth, the risk of zoonoses remains to be determined.

A few species of free-living amoeboids have been identified as zoonotic. Although these protozoans are not believed to have significant virulence, they are unable to replicate at the lower intestinal temperatures typically found in herps. In these cases reptiles may only be temporary hosts that facilitate the transmission of the protozoa to mammals. Furthermore, some amoeba cysts are very resistant in the environment and commonly carry pathogenic bacteria strains, which are zoonotic.[27] Assessment of the zoonotic status should play a role in the decision to treat any presumptive parasite, but should not be the sole deciding factor.

CLASSES OF PROTOZOAL GASTROINTESTINAL PARASITES

Protists, as a kingdom, have the unique description as being both a single cell and a complete organism at the same time. While this description is applicable, protozoal parasites still fit within the evolutionary description of a parasite as an organism that has lost some of its components that have allowed it to best adapt for success in its environment. Parasitic protozoa still require their hosts to survive, as most of them display specific tissue tropism within the gastrointestinal tract, many of them invade their host intracellularly, and, despite our lack of understanding of the specific mechanisms, require the unique environment provided by their host.

Although this is a list of "parasitic" protozoa, not all of these are confirmed as intrinsically pathogenic. As discussed earlier, treatment should be assessed on a case-by-case basis as virulence to any particular species is questioned. In addition, as much identification as possible should be performed to differentiate between parasites, possible parasites, and pseudoparasites. Protists that are considered nonvirulent (normal flora) may develop virulence with significant increases in population density/increased competition with other species of protozoa, so treatment (in the form of population reduction) may be indicated. Nor is this list all-inclusive; there are many additional protozoans that have possible virulence but very low significance.

Apicomplexa

Apicomplexan organisms are spore-forming protists that are obligate parasites of animals, often with high host specificity. Most of the protozoa within this group form an apicoplast (a cellular structure essential for the survival of the organism containing one) and an apical complex, used to enter the host cell.

Cryptosporidia

All *Cryptosporidium* organisms are obligate intracellular parasites of vertebrates that form highly environmentally resistant spores. This genera of organism has been documented as infecting not only all portions of the gastrointestinal tract but also the biliary and the respiratory tract.[28] In humans, they are split into the gastric group and the intestinal group.[29] This delineation seems to be somewhat applicable to herptile *Cryptosporidium*, with some species (*Cryptosporidium saurophila, Cryptosporidium varanii*) categorized as intestinal and others (*Cryptosporidium serpentes*) categorized as gastric. However, some species may be able to infect different reptilian species with differing tissue tropism, requiring either recategorization or additional categories, as applicable. Furthermore, infestations may present as either a carrier state or a clinical state, and the same host may have their state change because of extraneous factors. As many other species of reptiles have only recently been identified as having their own species of *Cryptosporidium*, categorization is as yet incomplete.[30,31] Infections, despite differences in hosts, species, and even specific pathology, do have some commonality: (1) any infested animal has the potential to pass large numbers of oocysts in their stools that are highly infective to other hosts; (2) treatment is often unrewarding, with no consistent successful treatment protocols; (3) infected individuals typically have a fatal outcome.

Cryptosporidium infection has been confirmed in a wide variety of reptilian species, across many different families (**Fig. 3**).[28,32,33] Turtles and tortoises feature in relatively few reports, but more recent examinations have demonstrated that there appears to be chelonia-specific species of this protist with significant differences in virulence.[30] A study found that rat snakes were not able to become infected with inoculations of *Cryptosporidium* species from a wide range of homoeothermic hosts (mice, camels, chickens, cattle, guinea pigs), but readily became infected through oral inoculation of samples obtained from several species of reptiles (turtle, chameleon, tortoise, snake, lizard). The same study also found marked differences in pathogenicity between 2 related genera of snakes (*Pituophus* and *Elaphe* (*Pantherophis*)) that were infected with *Cryptosporidium* from the same source host. The conclusion was that there were marked differences in virulence of the same strain of *Cryptosporidium* between different genera/species of snakes.[34] Despite only 2 currently accepted named species that infect reptiles,[35] with today's identification techniques and the knowledge there are likely multiple species of *Cryptosporidium* derived from these,[28,36] the source of this variation in virulence may be determined to be from different species/subspecies of parasite rather than a variation in susceptibility. It is hoped that further studies will elucidate this point.

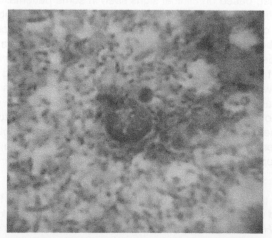

Fig. 3. *Cryptosporidium* sporocyst from a Leopard gecko (*Eublepharis macularius*) (acid-fast stain, original magnification ×1000). (*Courtesy of* A.K. Maas III, DVM, Bothell, WA.)

As stated, *Cryptosporidium* produced exceptionally environmentally resistant spores. Most available cleaning and disinfecting agents do not affect the viability these spores, and even quaternary ammonium compounds have, at best, fair results. The only confirmed methods to destroy environmental oocysts are 5% ammonia or 10% formalin with continuous wet contact of 18 hours above 4°C,[37] or with sufficient exposure to high-intensity ultraviolet radiation[38] (effective on both surfaces and in water). Studies have confirmed that neither chlorination nor ozonation of water will consistently destroy *Cryptosporidium* spores,[39,40] thus contamination is difficult to eliminate.

Cyclospora

Cyclospora, another spore-forming apicomplexan parasite, has been identified in a spotted desert racer (*Platyceps karelini*) with severe intestinal pathologic changes noted.[41] Although this parasite genera is considered a relatively new concern in human medicine and a significant emerging human disease,[42] there is very little in the herpetologic literature on this organism.

Coccidia

Coccidian parasites comprise a large group of intracellular protozoal parasites regularly found in reptiles. *Isospora* and *Eimeria* are well known genera from the mammalian literature, identified in carnivores, herbivores, and omnivores alike. Their prevalence in reptiles is similar, with identification in chelonians, snakes, and lizards, with possibly the best known in the herpetologic literature being *Isospora amphiboluri* from the inland bearded dragon (*Pogona vitticeps*) and the frilled lizard (*Chlamydosaurus kingii*).[43] With the exception of *Sarcocystis*, these parasites have a primarily direct life cycle. Like so many other protists, virulence seems to be related to protozoan parasite population density, host factors (stress, concomitant disease, and so forth), and, possibly, strain of the parasite, with both endogenous high and low virulence noted. When infected with a virulent strain/species, damage to the intestinal mucosa appears to be most common direct pathologic finding. This damage then leads to fluid loss, often associated with diarrhea, and hence chronic dehydration. The kidneys then are damaged by the chronic dehydration, leading to death from renal failure. A heat-labile neurotoxin produced by the parasite has been identified in bovine nervous coccidiosis.[44] Although no toxin has been identified in reptile forms, in the author's opinion it may exist, based on clinical signs seen in some patients.

Although *I amphiboluri* and other coccidia have been cited as being nonpathogenic, there are reports of disorders associated with infestation. Clinical condition and risk factors need to be assessed in each case. These parasites have indications that they may be moderately host specific, limited to possibly single or a few species of reptiles or at least within closely related genera. A report evaluating coccidian populations in a narrow geographic range within the Galapagos Islands found a species each of *Isospora* and *Eimeria* that were limited to inhabiting a single species of lizard, whereas other coccidians examined extended into other herpetologic species.[45] However, because coccidian organisms are so commonly an inhabitant of many animals, identification of actual parasites is important in being able to discern potential risks from pseudoparasites.[15]

Choleoeimeria

Choleoeimeria, a relatively recently identified coccidian, has been found in the gallbladders of veiled chameleons (*Chameleo calyptratus*),[46] Oustelet's chameleons (*Furcifur oustaleti*),[47] *Hemidactylus* geckos,[48] sandfish (*Scincus scincus scincus*),[49] and a legless lizard (*Amphisbaena alba*).[50] The hallmark of this particular coccidian is that it primarily infects that bile ducts and gallbladders of its host. This infection causes the invaded epithelial cells to hypertrophy and elevate above the surface, which leads to eventual obstruction of the tract. Most individuals identified with infections were found to have enlarged, dilated gallbladders that were difficult or impossible to express. Sporulated oocysts containing 4 sporozoites are readily identified within the feces of *Choleoeimeria*-infected animals, in contrast to only 2 sporozoites found in *Isospora* sp oocysts.

Caryospora

Caryospora, another coccidian found within the gastrointestinal tract of reptiles, has been associated with a death of an infected spitting cobra (*Naja nigricollis pallida*) and the severe morbidity of another.[51] Another report identified infected *Elaphe* species as being emaciated, but these animals also had concurrent infections with other parasites, and no histopathology was performed to confirm abnormality caused by the coccidian.[52] *Caryospora* has been identified in the intestinal tracts of many other snakes and lizards, but is not commonly associated with pathologic features. Thus, this coccidian is of low virulence and pathology and is only seen when there are additional, compounding, factors.

Intranuclear coccidiosis

Intranuclear coccidiosis is an emerging disease of tortoises that affects infected animals on a multisystemic basis. In addition to the respiratory, renal, reproductive, hemolymphatic, endocrine, and neurologic systems, these parasites have been found within the mucosa of the alimentary tract, liver, and pancreas.[19] Studies to assess susceptible species, routes of infection, and treatment options are currently under way. Antemortem diagnosis of this disease is particularly difficult in that oocysts are not believed to be passed in the stools.

Sarcocystis

Sarcocystis infections are reported in many species of reptiles, and appear to be almost equally described as both intermediate and definitive hosts.[53] *Sarcocystis* infections in the intermediate hosts are typically designated as an infection of muscle tissue. One report of this genera described encysting within the muscle of the tongue of a lizard. The diadem rat snake (*Spaelerosophis diademata*) was the first reptile found to be the definitive host of a *Sarcocystis* species, with abnormality developing within the lamina propria of the intestine. The lizard intermediate hosts, as expected, had their infections within muscle tissue.[54] A bull snake (*Pituophis melanoleucus sayi*) had developed anorexia for at least 1 month before death, and on histopathology necrosis of the esophagus and thickening of the proximal intestine with an inflammatory infiltrate were identified.[55] Other reptilian definitive hosts have since been identified. The genus *Besnoitia* has also been suggested as having reptilian definitive hosts, but on reclassification most of these protozoans have been incorporated into *Sarcocystis* and should be considered as such.

Mastigophora/Flagellates

Flagellates are all highly motile protozoans, by means of one or more flagella that provide propulsion. Some species may be mononucleate or binucleate, may have only anterior or both anterior and posterior flagella, can range from only 1 to 8 or more flagella, and may or may not have a membranous sail that assists them in mobility. Flagellate protozoa have many examples each of parasitic and commensal organisms from high to low virulence, transitory organisms as pseudoparasites, and free-living organisms that can also be found within fecal samples. Thus, accurate identification is necessary to make a diagnosis and develop an appropriate treatment plan.

Giardia

Giardia is a flagellated protozoan that is known to infect intestines across a wide range of vertebrate families and orders. Although there is one species that has been identified as the primary infection of humans (*Giardia lamblia*, also known as *Giardia intestinalis*, *Giardia duodenalis*), few, if any, orders of vertebrates are immune to infestation by this genera. Studies suggest that these protozoans may be more similar than other protists to higher eukaryotes.[56] Reptiles have been reported as a source of *Giardia muris* zoonotic infections,[57] but little is written regarding either this species or any other *Giardia* species in the herpetologic veterinary literature. It is commonly thought that *Giardia* may have low to no significant virulence in reptiles.[58]

Trichomonads

Trichomonads, including the genera *Trichomonas*, *Hexamastrix*, *Monocercomonas*, *Tetratricomonas*, *Tritrichomonas*, and others, are normally present in the gastrointestinal tract of many reptiles. Many species are known to have pathogenic characteristics, although their virulence has not been consistently shown. These organisms are suspected to cause abnormality extending as far back as even the fossil record. A fossilized *Tyrannosaurus rex* fossil skull was found to have lesions identified, consistent with classic oral osseous *Trichomonas* lesions seen in modern species.[59] Modern reptiles with trichomonads within their gastrointestinal tract have been identified with fibrinonecrotic enteritis[60] associated with polydipsia and polyuria (ie, increased production of fecal water). However, virulence cannot be considered equal among all strains of this parasite, let alone species or genera, as human infections of *Trichomonas vaginalis* have been identified with variable virulence depending on the specific strain present.[61] *Bothrops jararaca* was found to have an infestation of *Trichomonas* (morphologically similar to *Trichomonas acosta*) that was resolved with a single dose of metronidazole, 40 mg/kg orally.[62] No description was made in this case as to the virulence or disease present in the infected individual. *Monocercomonas* is widely distributed in a sample set of 182 snakes covering 23 genera. It was commonly noted that the protozoa were within the lamina propria and invaded the intestinal wall in 34 of the individuals examined.[63] Most commonly, however, variable degrees of enteritis have been the symptoms associated with virulence (**Figs. 4** and **5**),[64,65] although the presence of trichomonads within a fecal sample does not always constitute a

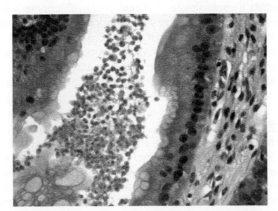

Fig. 4. Intestinal population of an unidentified flagellate protozoan in a leopard gecko (*E macularius*). Note changes present in mucosal epithelial cell height (hematoxylin-eosin [H&E] stain, original magnification ×400). (*Courtesy of* D. Reavill, DVM, West Sacramento, CA.)

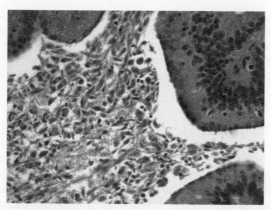

Fig. 5. Heavy intestinal population of an unidentified flagellate protozoan in a green anole (*Anolis carolinensis*). Note inflammatory cells migrating into mucosal epithelia (H&E stain, original magnification ×400). (*Courtesy of* D. Reavill, DVM, West Sacramento, CA.)

parasitic relationship.[66] A common belief in many cases such as this is that overproliferation of trichomonads is an indicator of an underlying condition, suboptimal husbandry, primary systemic infection, or other disease process that allows these organisms to increase their virulence.[67] Despite little clear evidence that many of the species have high virulence, when their hosts are immunosuppressed these protozoa seem capable of proliferating and causing pathologic disorder.

Hexamita
Hexamita, although having similar morphology to trichomonads and often mistaken as such, have been found to cause significant abnormality in reptiles. *Hexamita* has long been identified as a parasite of chelonians,[68] with pathologic changes confirmed in 8 different species. This genera has been described damaging the intestinal tract, and lesions and parasites have been found within other organs. Several species of both tortoises and turtles had *Hexamita parva* infestations of the bladder, kidneys, intestines, gallbladder, and liver, with significant abnormality identified in these organs.[69] Chelonia appear to have a greater susceptibility to renal infections, with marked damage to the kidney tissue developing from ascending infections through the ureters.[70] Signs of disease in infected individuals may be subtle, with hosts perhaps only displaying dilute, watery urine. Nephrosis often is a sequela of chronic infestations, developing into hyperparathyroidism as calcium regulation is lost because of the inability to metabolize active vitamin D. If not treated early and appropriately, death will often ensue. Although the species of the organisms were not identified, flagellated protozoans were identified to have invaded the pancreas via the pancreatic duct of snakes, as well as causing salpingitis following an infestation of the oviducts.[67] Invasion of the circulatory system has also been reported, with organisms present on blood film cytologies.[20] There are many more protozoal candidates that can be included in this class, including *Spironucleus*, *Leptomonas*, *Proteromonas*, and others.

Parabasalia
Parabasalia-class flagellates are also commonly identified in the gut of many reptiles, particularly insectivores. Several species of these have been found to be normal flora in the gut of tropical cockroaches[66] and are considered to be both a parasite of

insects[71] and a pseudoparasite within the reptiles that eat them. As they are commonly found in large numbers within fecal samples, it can be very easy to think them as a parasite of the herpetologic patient and be misdiagnosed. For this reason, it may be advisable to feed an insectivorous reptile that is suspected of having a parasitic infection a prepared insect-free diet for at least several days before fecal collection.

Rhizopoda/Amoeboids

Amoebae are a common finding in many reptilian gastrointestinal tracts, but are still poorly understood. It is most likely that most of these protozoal organisms are nonpathogenic, with very low endemic virulence, but there are a few individuals that have displayed an inherent high pathogenicity. These protists have a variable size and shape, with their mobility derived from the ability to form pseudopodia projections and "crawl" along them.

Entamoeba

Entamoeba invadens is the best documented as having significant virulence in reptiles. It has been identified in all orders of reptile, and confirmed in many genera. There may be some correlation suggesting that herbivorous species are more likely to be asymptomatic carriers, whereas carnivorous reptiles are more likely to have high endemic pathology.[70] These parasites can cause significant lesions in many squamates, developing membranous enteritis with inflammation and edema of the intestines (**Fig. 6**). The inflammation can easily develop into coelomic adhesions and mucosal erosions, and the parasite is known to invade the liver via the portal vein (**Fig. 7**). This invasion has been found to cause massive infarctions of the liver and subsequent death.[20] Furthermore, in snakes the most severe disorder has been found to occur when infected animals are kept at 25°C, compared with those kept at higher or lower temperatures,[72] suggesting that there is a temperature-sensitive pathologic action, possibly a cytotoxin.

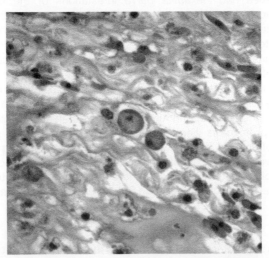

Fig. 6. Amoebic gastric infiltration of a common boa (*Boa constrictor* ssp) (H&E stain, original magnification ×400). (*Courtesy of* D. Reavill, DVM, West Sacramento, CA.)

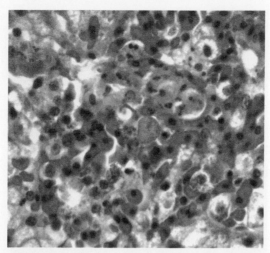

Fig. 7. Amoebic hepatic infiltration of a common boa (*Boa constrictor* ssp) (H&E stain, original magnification ×400). (*Courtesy of* D. Reavill, DVM, West Sacramento, CA.)

Blastocystis

Blastocystis has been identified within samples collected from the gastrointestinal tract in several reptiles, including lizards, snakes, a crocodile, and Chelonia.[73] Pathogenesis has been hotly debated but eventually confirmed in human *Blastocystis* infestations,[74] as well as the potential for infection in guinea pigs and other rodents; this creates the potential for both zoonoses and reverse zoonoses.[75] No reports, however, have provided evidence for significant virulence or abnormality in reptiles.

Ciliata

Ciliated protozoa are readily encountered in fecal samples from a wide range of reptilian hosts, and are readily identified by their smooth, sweeping motion precipitated by the short motile cilia on the surface of their cell membrane. Although individual cilia are not easily seen in fresh preparations, the hallmark wave-like appearance is the identifying feature of all of these organisms. Unlike most of the protists listed here, there is variation in size between species, with some ciliated protozoa being relatively large, up to 30 μm in length.

Balantidium

Balantidium is well known from both human and nonhuman primate literature and has been found in several reptile gastrointestinal tracts. Tortoises have multiple types and even large numbers of *Balantidium* present in their intestinal tract, but with little to no abnormality.[76] Further investigation has suggested that although most infestations are asymptomatic, this genus uses endogenously produced hyaluronidase to damage the intestinal mucosa (most commonly the colon) and penetrate the tissues, where they cause necrosis. Although tortoises with heavy infestations have been found with *Balantidium* organisms within the liver causing abscess formation,[70] this is likely an example of increased virulence as a result of increased population density.

Nyctotherus

Nyctotherus, another ciliate, is commonly found in many species of reptiles, particularly in tortoises and herbivorous lizards (**Fig. 8**). Large numbers of motile protozoa,

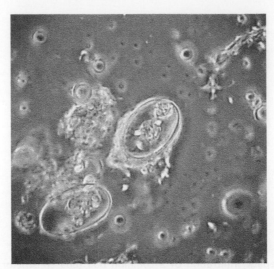

Fig. 8. Nyctotherium from a Russian tortoise (*Testudo horsfeldii*) (wet mount preparation, phase contrast, original magnification ×100). (*Courtesy of* A.K. Maas III, DVM, Bothell, WA.)

one type resembling *Nyctotherus* sp protozoa, were identified from fecal samples taken from Marlborough green geckos (*Naultinus manukanus*). These protozoa were also present in lesions within the lumen of the intestine of one animal post mortem on histopathology.[77] It can be surmised that there may have been high virulence factors potentially created by the competition of protozoa within this individual lizard, but there was no demonstration as to whether any or all of the protozoa seen were specifically responsible for the pathologic condition identified. Within samples from a colubrid snake, *Leptodeira maculata*, a new species of *Nyctotherus*, and another ciliate, *Zelleriella*, were identified, suggesting that carnivorous species of reptiles may also play host to these organisms. No abnormality in the snake was cited.[78]

Opalina

Opalina have been rarely identified within the gastrointestinal tract of reptiles, but no evidence of virulence has been reported. *Opalina* are most commonly associated with normal gastrointestinal flora of amphibians, and may be a pseudoparasite of reptiles derived from their diet.

Microsporidia

Microsporidia is a relatively recent addition to the list of reptilian gastrointestinal parasites. There is still much debate as to whether this particular organism is a protozoan or a fungus, but given the evidence that there are genetic characteristics of both groups, this organism is categorized herein as a protist. This parasite has been best characterized in the inland bearded dragon (*P vitticeps*),[79] with infections causing hepatic necrosis, granulomatous inflammation of the colon, adrenal glands, and ovaries. The life cycle is still being studied, but transmission has been linked to ingestion of infected crickets.[67] Organisms have also been found within cells of the lung, stomach, and brain. Reptilian microsporidia have recently undergone nucleic acid analysis showing very high sequence similarity to the rabbit form of *Encephalitozoon cuniculi* (Fig. 9).[80]

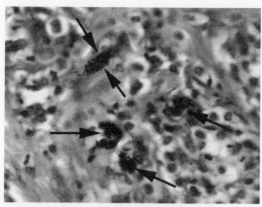

Fig. 9. Microsporidia in the colonic submucosa of a bearded dragon (*Pogona vitticeps*). Note extensive inflammation present (*arrows*) (Gram stain, original magnification ×1000). (*Courtesy of* Elliott Jacobson, DVM, PhD, Gainesville, FL.)

APPLICATIONS
Identification Options

The most commonly used technique for identification of gastrointestinal protozoal parasites is light microscopy. This modality is particularly useful in that almost all veterinary practices have a microscope, and the isolating/identifying techniques have a relatively short learning curve. The basic equipment necessary for analysis and identification should comprise a compound microscope with a self-contained light source, a mechanical stage, an iris diaphragm with vertical adjustment, and multiple objectives including at least a 10×, 40× (dry), and 100× oil immersion. Contrast-enhancing equipment such as differential interference contrast, dark-field, and phase-contrast should be seriously considered, as they allow for much easier and more accurate identification of protozoa as well as dramatically increasing the proficiency of the operator (**Fig. 10**). Adding a binocular head, multiple-power eyepieces, and additional objectives (particularly 4× and 20×) are all helpful, but not necessary. Supplies necessary for isolation, including stains, are listed below and may depend on the protozoa to be identified.

The most common fecal analysis technique performed in other species is a simple sugar/sulfate flotation, but this technique has significant limitations as regards identification of reptile protozoans. This method is generally poor for identifying flagellated protozoa, in that much of the identification of this class requires either live organisms or high-power stained microscopy to allow for direct visualization of flagellar structures. However, it is very effective for isolating coccidian species (*Isospora* and *Eimeria*, in particular), allowing identification and categorization, but is a very challenging method for identifying *Cryptosporidia*. *Nyctotherus* ciliate cysts are relatively large for a protozoal cyst and are identified on flotation preparations. No known reports are available for identification of microsporidia organisms using flotation techniques.

Direct (wet or native) mount fecal analysis is another simple technique that has high-yield results for identification of many classes of protozoal organisms. Depending on the host and the parasite, direct visualization of the parasites can be achieved with oral swabs, fecal samples, cloacal washes, gastric aspirates, and almost any sample collected from the gastrointestinal tract. Very fresh samples are best, as flagellated, ciliated, and amoebic parasites will generally become immobile within 10 to 20 minutes of defecation/collection. Inactivity will occur almost immediately on refrigeration,

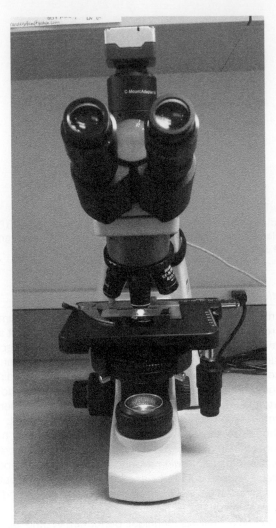

Fig. 10. A typical high-quality microscope with optimizations for parasitic identification. Note the trinocular head with a digital camera for both shared observation and recording of images; 4×, 10×, 20×, 40×, and 100× (oil immersion) objectives; precision mechanical stage; and a diaphragm containing filters both for bright-field and phase-contrast microscopy. (*Courtesy of* A.K. Maas III, Bothell, WA.)

making identification challenging to impossible. Oocysts of flagellates, ciliates, and cryptosporidia may also be present, but can be difficult to identify unless they occur within the sample in large numbers and are reviewed by an experienced microscopist. It is important to note the numbers and location of flagella, flagella-associated structures, size and number of nuclei, motion pattern, and all other physical characteristics of motile parasites so that identification can be confirmed for an estimate of virulence and, thus, a determination to treat (**Fig. 11**).

A stained dry-slide preparation is a useful method to both identify infections and confirm the taxonomy of a specific protozoal parasite. Microscope slides are typically prepped from a fecal sample mixed with saline to distribute and thin the material,

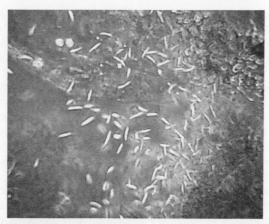

Fig. 11. Hexamita-class protozoa from a bearded dragon (*Pogona vitticeps*) (wet mount fecal preparation, phase contrast, original magnification ×100). (*Courtesy of* A.K. Maas III, DVM, Bothell, WA.)

which can then be directly mounted, filtered and then mounted, or centrifuged and then mounted. After drying, several staining techniques can be used to define protozoan cellular structures and enhance visualization of the parasite or its oocyst.

Flagellated and ciliated protozoa can be well visualized using these techniques. Textbooks of parasitology and journals, as well as Web sites,[81] have excellent stained photomicrographs to aid in the identification of genera, so a discussion of the physical characteristics of each protozoan is not necessary here. However, specific knowledge of the natural history of the host is necessary with many of the classes of protists to identify down to a species level. Common staining techniques such as Wright stain and modified Romanowski staining work well for most protozoal organisms. Alternative staining methods and parasite-specific techniques are discussed here.

Amoeboid organisms can be particularly difficult to identify by microscopy. Direct mount analysis can be particularly useful for a quick and simple diagnosis, but in the author's opinion trophozoites are rarely identified on wet mount preparations, and typically stay active for only a short time after defecation. Cysts, although they may be present on a direct sample, can be few in number and difficult to identify. Sedimentation-concentrating methods are typically used to concentrate the oocysts, improved by centrifugation. Special staining (eg, Wheatley-Trichrome, Eosin-Y) techniques to identify amoebic trophozoites under high-powered microscopy are common methods in human medicine. The most common staining techniques used for amoeboid identification are iodine-stained preparations[82] and periodic acid-Schiff (PAS) staining, both of which make the organism distinct from the ground material under light microscopy. A commercially available monoclonal antibody to *Entamoeba histolytica* has been used with good success in samples from ball pythons (*Python regius*) believed to be infected with *E invadens*.[83]

Acid-fast (there are several methods commonly used, eg, Ziehl-Neelsen) staining methods are advised for the identification of microsporidia and cryptosporidia. These organisms stain a distinctive magenta color with this technique while the background material typically turns a medium purple-blue color. The microscopist must still be familiar with the physical characteristics of these organisms because, although there are few other structures that will stain positive with acid-fast techniques (primarily including, but not limited to, *Mycobacterium*, anaerobic spore-forming bacilli, some flagellated protozoan oocysts, and sperm), there is still the possibility of misidentification. It must be remembered, however, that mammalian species of *Cryptosporidium* are not infective to reptiles, so if there is the possibility of the ingestion of an infected prey item, positive acid-fast cytology should not automatically be interpreted as an infected host.

Intranuclear coccidiosis, as mentioned earlier, has been particularly difficult to diagnose ante mortem. However, it has been found that these organisms may be prevalent in the sinuses of infected individuals and can be identified cytologically from both smears and sinus biopsies. In addition to being morphologically identifiable using a modified Wright-Giemsa stain, they also stain positive with PAS and acid-fast techniques.[84] To prevent misdiagnosis, however, all suspect cases should be confirmed with polymerase chain reaction (PCR) identification.

PCR testing is the amplification and identification of specific nucleic acid sequences to aid in the identification of organisms present within a sample, and is becoming much more commonplace in veterinary medicine. With protozoal parasites, pathogens present can be identified or confirmed, often from a simple fecal sample. Furthermore, this technique can also be used to confirm infestation from a tissue sample. With this method species identification is the norm, but many tests available can be used as a broad-range search for genera identification when a species is not well understood or known.

The PCR technique is available to aid in diagnosing protozoal infestation from commercial laboratories, universities, and government testing laboratories. These techniques can be useful in both identifying occult infections and confirming symptomatic disease, but the specific test performed should be researched before use, because some of the tests may be species specific and may allow for a missed diagnosis, whereas others may provide sequencing for a more thorough examination but can be prohibitively expensive and take weeks to produce results. The specificity and accuracy of any PCR test can vary with the probes used, so an understanding of the method used is essential to responsibly selecting a test to be performed.

Giardia and *Cryptosporidium* are commonly identified by PCR in human medicine. The primers used in human medicine to identify *Cryptosporidium* target the small subunit ribosomal RNA,[85] the oocyst wall protein,[86] or other specific genetic markers. Similarly, human medical PCR targets the small subunit ribosomal RNA[87] for *Giardia* identification, but also the glutamate dehydrogenase gene.[88] In veterinary diagnostics, the 18S ribosomal RNA gene is the most commonly used target sequence for both of these organisms, and has allowed for the differentiation of possible new species.[89] Moreover, PCR analysis has been confirmed as a reliable, accurate, and sensitive method to identify cryptosporidia in stool samples[90] as well as in gastric contents or regurgitant.[91] In published articles, PCR amplification has also been an excellent method for identification of infections containing multiple species of *Cryptosporidium* within the same host,[89] and to aid in the identification of new species.[92]

PCR testing for *Entamoeba* is also becoming available, but few laboratories are offering it owing to limited demand. To the author's knowledge, *E invadens* analysis is the only commercially available test at present.[93] Only large institutions offer the ability to explore both amoeboid and flagellate (non-*Giardia*) infestations,[63] and then only use more laborious PCR-sequencing techniques. Owing to the paucity of literature with clear understanding regarding these families of infestations, even this method may have limitations regarding analysis. No known commercially available PCR is currently available for ciliate identification.

Antibody titers can be an effective means of tracking infection response, but not an effective means to diagnose acute infections. Because the body must have time following exposure to generate antibodies, paired titers must be used to demonstrate an increase in antibody production to a specific antigen. This test may also be an effective method to determine a negative infection status, provided it is performed sequentially at appropriate intervals to provide data. At present, *Giardia* titers are available for both humans and domestic pets, but no tests have been validated for use in the herptile patient.

Biopsy and histopathology have long been considered the gold standard to determine infections of many, if not all, protozoal parasites. The advantage to these methods is that they allow for specific demonstration of infection and assessment of inflammatory processes present, lesions associated with the parasite, and a complete evaluation of multiple organ systems that the parasite may be affecting or infecting. The disadvantage is obvious in that these procedures require invasive procedures that impart risk to the patient, and it is difficult, if not impossible, to acquire samples from all tissues (ie, cardiac, brain) in an antemortem patient.

After processing of the samples, they may be evaluated using one or more of many different methods to further assist in identification. Any of the aforementioned staining methods may be used to provide general determination of organisms present and the condition of associated tissues (eg, hematoxylin-eosin, Wright/Giemsa, Romanowsky), or more specialized staining processes that selectively stain parasites based on the structure and stain-binding properties (eg, PAS, acid-fast, trichrome). Knowledge of the mechanisms of each of these staining protocols is essential in understanding the limitation of diagnoses and preventing overinterpretation of observed findings. For example, gastric biopsies have been found to have good sensitivity and 100% specificity when diagnosing *Cryptosporidium* in snakes.[94] Although the presence of this organism may be confirmed and associated with pathologic lesions also identified, speciation of the parasite found is difficult to impossible without additional testing, and this is reflected by nearly all protozoan parasites.

Immunofluorescent antibodies (IFA) have been used and studied to improve the accuracy of diagnoses made from biopsy samples and histopathologic review. This method uses purified antibodies to parasitic epitopes that are conjugated to a secondary molecule for stain enhancement following binding to the thin sections. This system is hampered by many aspects, including difficulty of generation of specific antibodies, requirements for extensive validation, difficulty in repeatability, and significant issues with cross-reactivity with other cells, and thus has fallen out of favor, with a preference for other methods as they have become available. Although this technique is regularly used in a laboratory setting and sometimes in human medicine, protozoal identification using IFA methods in herpetologic medicine appears to be unavailable except as a research technique.

In situ hybridization of histopathologic samples is an excellent means to confirm diagnoses. This procedure uses a known segment of genetic sequence as a probe linked to a secondary molecule that is used to facilitate a reaction that permits identification (ie, radioassay, fluorescence, horseradish peroxidase staining, and so forth) of the specific organism. This testing method has higher specificity and sensitivity than IFA testing, but like IFA also requires extensive testing to validate the specific probe used. Unfortunately, there are no known commercially available tests for the herptile patient, and they can only be performed through research universities at this time. Validated tests have been performed in an amoeboid, flagellate, and *Cryptosporidium* species, but it is not known whether there may be cross-reactivity with closely related parasite species.[63] To assess this, extensive research still needs to be performed to not only identify other species of the target parasite, but also compare target sequences and design species-specific probes and techniques.

HOW CAN VIRULENCE BE DETERMINED? (IS THIS A PROBLEM THAT NEEDS TO BE TREATED?)

It has been mentioned many times throughout this article that virulence needs to be assessed as a means to determine if treatment is necessary. However, there is little concrete evidence regarding how to assess virulence. The most commonly used mechanism is that of clinical presentation, but at the same time this method is the most subjective and the most fraught with error in the herptile patient. These animals are particularly stoic in general, and with very few pathognomonic signs it is nearly impossible for the clinician to determine, based on clinical presentation, whether a reptile's protozoal inhabitants are causing the symptoms commonly seen.

Degrees of depression are commonly seen with protozoal parasitism, but is a symptom seen with almost any reptilian disease. Neurologic signs can be primary or secondary symptoms, depending on whether the parasite is directly affecting the central nervous system or causing other metabolic dyscrasias. Microsporidia and intranuclear coccidiosis are known to infect the brain and cause direct central nervous system symptoms, ranging from depression and weakness to ataxia, seizures, and death. *Hexamita* have been found in blood smears of infected reptiles, and theoretically could develop into parasitic meningitis and encephalitis. Reptiles with very heavy coccidial infections are not uncommonly seen by the author to have neurologic symptoms that resolve with treatment, anecdotally supporting the concept that they may have the capacity for producing neurotoxins as seen in other species.

Anorexia is possibly the most common symptom seen with protozoal parasitism. It must be remembered that anorexia is a symptom, not a disease, and needs to be considered as such. However, it is possibly the most common symptom seen in virtually any reptile malaise, so there can be no specific association with parasitism. When associated with parasite infections it often will resolve with treatment, which may extend to several months.

Observation of specific symptoms determined as being associated with gastrointestinal disease can be used as supportive evidence. Diarrhea is possibly the most commonly seen symptom, but subjective assessment will help provide more information about the condition. Mucus production increases with parasite-induced abnormality, and sometimes the entire stool become encased in a sheath of mucus. Blood is rarely seen in stools, but when it is, parasitic infestation by *Entamoeba* species should be considered. Other changes in stools may occur with protozoal parasitism. Reptiles may pass undigested food in their feces, and many species of herbivorous reptiles will have their stools develop a stronger, foul odor when the host develops a case of parasitism.

Gastrointestinal functional changes are not uncommon with protozoal infections. Regurgitation can occur with *C serpentes* infections in snakes, whereas diarrhea is associated with *Cryptosporidium saurium* in leopard geckos (*Eublepharis macularius*); this difference in symptoms is due to the different tissue tropism of the different species of parasite. With other parasites, both hypomotility (constipation) and hypermotility (diarrhea) can be seen, and it is the changes in motility rather than one or the other that can be associated with virulence.

Dehydration, as discussed earlier, is a nonspecific secondary sign, but when it occurs with gastrointestinal symptoms in the presence of possibly virulent protozoa it needs to be addressed and corrected.

Other symptoms may vary depending on the species of both host and parasite. The author has seen many cases of gingivitis and oral disease in bearded dragons (*P *vitticeps*) infected with *Trichomonas*, but not ocular disease. By contrast, leopard geckoes (*E macularius*) with *Trichomonas* infections are often seen to have conjunctivitis, with parasites identified in the conjunctival sac. Granted, there is a high likelihood of different species, and even genera, of protozoa infecting the different hosts, but this comparison elucidates the need for examining specific symptoms to determine significance and virulence.

As discussed earlier, single specific laboratory testing (complete blood cell count, serum chemistries, protein electrophoresis) other than the specific parasite testing described may or may not assist the clinician in assessing virulence of an infection. However, serial testing of any of these diagnostic methods may significantly improve the interpretation of obtained results, as changes often can be seen over time, concurrent to treatment, and as the patient recovers. The greatest limiting factor is the limited laboratory diagnostic testing options available (eg, poor availability of biliverdin testing rather than bilirubin tests currently available) to the herptile patient. It is the author's hope that as the knowledge base continues to expand, more tests will become available.

Imaging the patient can be of assistance in certain protozoal infections. Coelomic ultrasonography can assist in the diagnosis of *Choleoeimeria* by identifying enlarged gall bladders, thickened bile duct walls, and possible obstructions. Thickened intestinal walls may help assess virulence of other protozoal infestations. Radiographs or computed tomography might prove useful in evaluating bone loss or fistula formation in the sinuses of tortoises with intranuclear coccidiosis, and specifically identifying bone loss in jaws as a result of *Trichomonas* infections and abscesses.

Bacterial culture and sensitivity testing may be useful in determining parasitic virulence, but also should be considered to determine whether there are coinfections with or superinfections caused by pathogenic bacteria. Unfortunately, many species of bacteria typically associated with pathologic conditions in other classes of vertebrates are considered to be normal flora in reptiles. Similar to assessing protozoal virulence, the difficulty lies in determining whether species identified on culture techniques are the source of disease seen, rather than an incidental finding or normal gastrointestinal flora. Adding to this problem is the limitation of culture techniques and a very limited knowledge of growth requirements of bacteria inhabiting poikilotherms. Studies examining gastrointestinal flora of American alligators (*Alligator alligator*) using PCR technology identified at least 10^3 additional species of bacteria that were unable to be cultured using routine systems (D. Gillespie, PhD, personal communication, 2001). This finding suggests that there could be multitudes of bacterial pathogens playing a role in reptile gastrointestinal disease that we are unable to identify.

Even with testing of the patient to determine the presence of protists, and additional diagnostics to assess both local and systemic effects and identification of coinfections, determination of virulence can still be difficult. Key to this is data supporting what constitutes a "normal" population for the host species what "normal" levels should be for each particular protozoan. Unfortunately, such knowledge has yet to be determined. Therefore, a subjective assessment of protozoal counts needs to be made in every case of potential parasitism. Owing to a dearth of published information, this is best done once the clinician has reviewed many samples from a large number of individuals and is experienced in assessing protozoal species, superinfections, and densities in a wide range of reptile hosts. Until more studies are performed, subjective experience is still the best resource.

Lastly, the need to assess the significance of captive husbandry versus wild natural history has to be considered. There can be no argument that reptiles in their native environment are host to many parasites, often with low virulence. Even with "perfect" environmental factors, they occasionally succumb to parasite loads. With the additive stresses placed on a host in captivity, it should be no surprise that reptiles in collections commonly are affected by protozoans that generally are considered to have no to low virulence in free-ranging individuals. Thus, 2 conclusions can be made: (1) if a protist is known to have innate pathogenicity in wild populations, it should be treated in captive animals; and (2) if a host is displaying symptoms that an inhabitant protist has indications of virulence, it should be treated in captive animals.

TREATMENT

Although this section's purpose is to cover therapeutics, it must be borne in mind that before treatment can occur, a plan must be organized. The first step, as discussed earlier, is to determine the type of parasite present, preferably identifying at least to a genus level so that one can obtain at least a coarse assessment of the risk present. Second, the virulence needs to be determined, so that a need for treatment is confirmed. Third, knowledge of the parasite's life cycle, including but not limited to mechanisms of infection, generation time, host range and stages, tissue tropism, and stability in the environment, all need to be considered when designing a specific treatment plan. Fourth, treatment options need to be reviewed, taking into consideration the sensitivities of the protist as well as safety to the host. This plan also needs to consider underlying or secondary conditions and their treatment as applicable, to ensure that the host has the best chance possible for recovery. Fifth, sanitation of the environment and elimination of the parasite source must be carried out to prevent occurrence of a recrudescence or reinfection. Lastly, a plan for confirming either reduction of the parasite to an acceptable level or elimination (and determining which is most appropriate) must be decided upon and initiated. As related herein, treatment is not merely the dosing of medication to the host, but rather an integral process of all the aforementioned topics.

Therapeutic agents for reptiles, however, are fairly limited in scope. Unsurprisingly there are no US Department of Agriculture–labeled drugs available for use in reptile species, let alone any labeled antiparasitics. Most compounds have undergone no pharmacokinetic studies and, with few safety studies published, they are used empirically based on information carried from domestic companion animal medicine, anecdotal successes, and a handful of published reports. New drugs, both those listed here and otherwise, are constantly being tried, but the clinician should know that even less is known of the effects of these compounds on herptile species, and especially that an effective, safe use in one species may have little bearing on another.

This section is not intended to be an exhaustive list of therapeutics or protocols available to the reptile practitioner for use in cases addressing protozoal parasitism. Knowledge of the general function and interactions of any therapeutic is the basis of good medicine. References for this are available in both the human[95] and veterinary[96] literature, and should be reviewed before use.[97] For medications and doses that pertain specifically to reptile parasite therapy, there are excellent lists and texts in print that provide such data.[98,99] These lists cannot be used indiscriminately, as these are simply listings of treatments from publications and, as stated in a disclaimer in one of them, "…the authors do not necessarily endorse specific products, procedures or dosages reported in this book."[100] Any clinician using these texts needs to consider the purpose for choosing a medication, the clinical presentation of the patient, possible secondary and/or adverse effects, and the specific physiology of the affected species.

It is strongly encouraged for each and every clinician to research and read (in advance, ideally) the references cited in these texts pertaining to reptile medicine not only for each medication but also for each dose and application listed. The knowledge and understanding of these citations are essential for both appropriate treatment and a successful outcome. With the paucity of blinded clinical trials and pharmacokinetic studies in addition to the enormous range of species encountered in practice, ultimately the decision of how to treat lies entirely with the clinician. The best possible outcome will be thus produced by the fullest application of evidence-based-medicine. In other words, in those cases where data and evidence may be scarce, the clinician needs to take all available data and apply them to best possible effect. Simply put, when there is no specific standardized protocol, the final decision to treat must be clearly justifiable based on the available information.

Specific Treatment Considerations

Treatment using metronidazole or related compounds is the most common therapy available for most protozoal parasites. This class of medication has been found to be effective for flagellates, ciliates, and amoeboid parasites. However, anecdotal reports exist of drug resistance or failure to clear the parasites with therapy with even repeat courses of nitroimidazole-class drugs in reptiles, so changing specific drugs may be beneficial. *Trichomonas gallinae* has been reported to have differing levels of drug resistance within different clonal isolates of the same strain of parasite,[101] so retesting for the presence of the parasite is necessary, followed by alternative therapeutic options. Many different dosing strategies are available for reptile patients, with some validated by pharmacokinetics.[102,103]

Combinatorial therapy consisting of metronidazole and doxycycline has been circulating in discussions for treatment of amoebiasis in reptiles. One source indicated that combinatorial use has been effective in controlling clinical balantidiosis, suggesting a use in cases of ciliate overgrowth.[70] However, no references were found against *Entamoeba*, and it is suspected by the author that the doxycycline is being used based on this reference plus efficacy of treatment of protozoal parasitism (ciliates) in fish[104] and poultry (flagellates).[105] If improvement is seen with this protocol in reptiles, it is suspected that it is a result of control of secondary infections associated with intestinal lesions caused by *Entamoeba*, as there is no reported efficacy of this drug against *Sarcodina* class organisms.

Tortoises with *Hexamita* infestations present a unique challenge for dosing, as successfully administering the same animal twice in a row is often not possible. Particularly for smaller patients, soaking tortoises in a 1-g/L solution of ronidazole, 30 minutes once daily for 18 days, has been found to be effective at clearing hexamitiasis (K. Wright, DVM, DABVP, personal communication, 2013).

Paromomycin, 50 to 75 mg/kg orally, once daily for 21 days, has been used with success by the author in cases of resistant flagellated protozoal strains. The specific dose needs to be adjusted based on the condition and physiology of the patient, and has little to do with the severity of infection.

Toltrazuril and ponazuril are recent additions to the arsenal for the treatment of protozoal parasites. Ponazuril has been found to be particularly effective for the treatment of *Isospora* spp in infected bearded dragons.[106] Despite their being the most commonly used therapy for coccidian infestations, sulfa drugs are known to be nephrotoxic, particularly in cases of dehydration. Reptiles' renal systems may be concentrating sulfa compounds in their nephrons, potentially further increasing toxicities of these drugs and increasing the risk of renal failure. Toltrazuril and ponazuril therefore are much safer choices in reptiles infected with parasites known to cause significant dehydration, as these are not known to have renal toxicity.

Toltrazuril has also been evaluated as an effective therapy for the treatment of *Isospora jaracimrrmani* in *Chameleo calyptratus*, but not in treatment of *Choleoeimeria*.[107] The difference in efficacy of this compound between 2 species of coccidian may be due to variation in sensitivity of the organisms to the medication, but is more likely due to toltrazuril's efficacy, concentration, or modification within the gallbladder, and further studies are needed to elucidate this. It has been suggested to use sulfonamides for the treatment of *Choleoeimeria*, but even these may not always be effective.[70]

Therapy using a commercially available moxidectin/imidialoprid preparation has been examined in an effort to eliminate *I amphiboluri* parasites in both bearded dragons (*P vitticeps*) and frilled lizards (*C kingii*), but was not found to be effective.[108]

Treatment of intranuclear coccidiosis using toltrazuril has been used with success, with pulsatile dosing at 15 mg/kg.[109] Based on the success using this compound, it is also suspected that ponazuril would also be successful because of its shared metabolic pathways, although no published data exist at this time (P. Gibbon, DVM, DABVP, personal communications, 2011).

Fenbendazole is a commonly used anthelmintic, but has been found to have efficacy in treating *Giardia* infections in mammals through inhibition of β-tubulin pathways.[110] Studies have shown that fenbendazole has higher efficacy than other benzimidazole-class drugs in antiprotozoal effects,[111] but little efficacy against *Trichomonas* or *Entamoeba*. As *Giardia* is of little clinical concern in herpetologic protozoal infections, this therapeutic may not have significant value in these cases.

Amoebic infections may be successfully treated with metronidazole or ronidazole, but are more likely to have treatment failures, as these compounds are only effective against the trophozoite forms. Paromomycin or iodoquinol are often more successful because they are also effective against the cyst form. Either of these may also be used alone or in combination with a nitroimidazole for combinatorial effect. Again, the condition and specific physiology of the patient should form the basis for a therapy chosen.

Cryptosporidium remains the greatest treatment challenge in veterinary parasitology today. As stated earlier, this organism is extremely durable in the environment, and despite a plethora of attempts at pharmacologic control, at present there seems to be no effective cure or means of elimination in the reptile patient.

Nitroimidazoles have been tried, but not found to be effective in cases of *Cryptosporidium* infections, although they appear to be able to temporarily reduce shedding of cysts. Thus, if accurate diagnostics are to be made on a patient, one must be certain to discontinue all medications for at least 14 days before collecting samples for testing. Paromomycin therapy has also been examined, with a significant reduction in both clinical signs and shedding of cysts at 100 mg/kg orally, although no elimination of the parasite could be confirmed.[112] Even at much higher doses (up to 800 mg/kg daily), clearance of the parasite could not be attained.[113]

Nitazoxanide is a relatively new drug to be used in cases of parasitism, with the bulk of studies showing that it has moderate to very good efficacy against a wide range of parasites (flukes, tapeworms, ascarids, protists) in humans.[114] Although it is the only drug approved by the Food and Drug Administration for use against cryptosporidiosis in humans in the United States, it has not found great success for controlling this disease in calves.[115] Preliminary studies in reptiles have found that it may be toxic in snakes with clinical disease at any dosage, although it may be effective (with safety unknown) against *Cryptosporidium* in leopard geckos (*E macularius*).[116]

Salicylhydroxamic acid (SHAM) has been shown to inhibit growth of *Cryptosporidium parvum* in in vitro conditions at up to 90% physiologic concentrations, in comparison with paromomycin only inhibiting growth at 20% at similar physiologic concentrations.[117] This inhibition is achieved by a novel approach of affecting the recently discovered alternate oxidase (AOX) pathway, a metabolic mechanism not found in vertebrate cells but also identified in *Toxoplasma* and *Plasmodium* spp; although this particular compound may not be the "holy grail" of *Cryptosporidium* treatment, it shows that there is great potential using novel mechanisms only now beginning to be understood.[118] Ascofuranone, an antibiotic and antineoplastic agent that has been found to have AOX-inhibiting function, has been shown to have efficacy in controlling *Trypanosoma brucei*,[119] with indications that it may be similarly effective against *Cryptosporidium*.[120]

SUMMARY

Ironically, protozoal parasites are some of the simplest organisms on the planet, having an already singular structure reduced down to less by the discarding of functions replaced by their host, but one of the most difficult to understand. Furthermore, the addition of these parasites into the poorly understood reptilian physiology only confounds efforts to formulate treatment plans when it is not completely clear when "a parasite" is indeed a parasite.

However, understanding this concept is key to deciding when and how to treat, and formulating the goals of treatment. In every case the parasite needs to be identified, an assessment of virulence made, the chosen therapeutic assessed and reviewed, and a comprehensive treatment plan decided upon that entails all aspects of the host. Only through this approach will appropriate and accurate herpetologic medicine be promoted and practiced.

IN MEMORIAM

This article is dedicated to my colleague, collaborator, teacher, dear friend, and partner in crime, Dr Kevin M. Wright, DVM, DABVP (Reptile and Amphibian Practice). His memory guided and motivated me in every word written, and I hope this is testament to his brilliance and the legacy he left behind in all of us who practice herptile medicine.

REFERENCES

1. Zimmer C. Parasite Rex. New York: Free Press; 2011. p. 126.
2. Taylor EW, Thomas JN. Membrane (contact) digestion in the three species of tapeworm *Hymenolepis diminuta*, *Hymenolepis microstoma* and *Moniezia expansa*. Parasitology 1968;58(3):535–46.
3. Hindsbo O, Andreassen J, Ruitenberg J. Immunological and histopathological reactions of the rat against the tapeworm *Hymenolepis diminuta* and the effects of anti-thymocyte serum. Parasite Immunol 1982;4(1):59–76.
4. Phares CK, Carroll RM. A lipogenic effect in intact male hamsters infected with plerocercoids of the tapeworm, *Spirometra mansonoides*. J Parasitol 1977;63: 690–3.
5. Salem MA, Phares CK. In vitro insulin-like actions of the growth factor from the tapeworm, *Spirometra mansonoides*. Proc Soc Exp Biol Med 1989;190(2): 203–10. Royal Society of Medicine.
6. Pai A, Yan G. Effects of tapeworm infection on male reproductive success and mating vigor in the red flour beetle, *Tribolium castaneum*. J Parasitol 2003;89(3): 516–21.

7. Carter V, Pierce R, Dufour S, et al. The tapeworm *Ligula intestinalis* (Cestoda: *Pseudophyllidea*) inhibits LH expression and puberty in its teleost host, *Rutilus rutilus*. Reproduction 2005;130(6):939–45.

8. Barber I, Hoare D, Krause J. Effects of parasites on fish behaviour: a review and evolutionary perspective. Rev Fish Biol Fish 2000;10:131–65.

9. Merino S, Moreno J, Sanz J, et al. Are avian blood parasites pathogenic in the wild? A medication experiment in blue tits (*Parus caeruleus*). Proc Biol Sci 2000; 267(1461):2507–10.

10. Bashey F, Morran LT, Lively CM. Co-infection, kin selection, and the rate of host exploitation by a parasitic nematode. Evol Ecol Res 2007;9(6):947–58.

11. Cox FE. Concomitant infections, parasites and immune responses. Parasitology 2001;122:S23–38.

12. Jacobson ER, Kopit W, Kennedy FA, et al. Coinfection of a bearded dragon, *Pogona vitticeps*, with adenovirus-and dependovirus-like viruses. Vet Pathol 1996; 33(3):343–6.

13. Dipineto L, Capasso M, Maurelli M, et al. Survey of co-infection by *Salmonella* and oxyurids in tortoises. BMC Vet Res 2012;8(1):69.

14. Carvalho AL, Deane MP. *Trypanosomatidae* isolated from *Zelus leucogrammus* (Perty, 1834) (Hemiptera, *Reduviidae*), with a discussion on flagellates of insectivorous bugs. J Eukaryot Microbiol 1974;21(1):5–8.

15. Berto BP, Lopes BDB, Flausino W, et al. Contribution on the study of *Isospora hemidactyli* Carini, 1936 and a report of an adeleid pseudoparasite of the house gecko *Hemidactylus mabouia*, from the Rio de Janeiro Metropolitan Region, Brazil. Rev Bras Parasitol Vet 2008;17(3):150–4.

16. Mitchell MA, Diaz-Figueroa O. Clinical reptile gastroenterology. Veterinary Clin North Am Exot Anim Pract 2005;8(2):277–98.

17. Evans HC, Elliot SL, Hughes DP. Hidden diversity behind the zombie-ant fungus *Ophiocordyceps unilateralis*: four new species described from carpenter ants in Minas Gerais, Brazil. PLoS One 2011;6(3):e17024.

18. Webster JP. The effect of *Toxoplasma gondii* on animal behavior: playing cat and mouse. Schizophr Bull 2007;33(3):752–6.

19. Garner MM, Gardiner CH, Wellehan JFX, et al. Intranuclear coccidiosis in tortoises: nine cases. Vet Pathol 2006;43(3):311–20.

20. Reichenbach-Klinke H, Elkan E. The principal diseases of lower vertebrates. New York: Academic Press; 1965. p. 399–420.

21. Broadhurst MJ, Ardeshir A, Kanwar B, et al. Therapeutic helminth infection of macaques with idiopathic chronic diarrhea alters the inflammatory signature and mucosal microbiota of the colon. PLoS Pathog 2012;8(11):e1003000.

22. Lafferty KD. Foraging on prey that are modified by parasites. Am Nat 1992; 140(5):854–67.

23. Gurgel ACF, Sartori ADS, De Araújo FAP. Protozoan parasites in captive chinchillas (*Chinchilla lanigera*) raised in the State of Rio Grande do Sul, Brazil. Parasitol Latinoam 2005;60:186–8 FLAP.

24. Frank SA. Models of parasite virulence. Q Rev Biol 1996;71(1):37–78.

25. Monis PT, Thompson RC. *Cryptosporidium* and *Giardia*-zoonoses: fact or fiction? Infect Genet Evol 2003;3(4):233–44.

26. Xiao L, Fayer R. Molecular characterisation of species and genotypes of *Cryptosporidium* and *Giardia* and assessment of zoonotic transmission. Int J Parasitol 2008;38(11):1239–55.

27. Schneller P, Pantchev N. Parasitology in snakes, lizards and chelonians. Frankfurt am Maim (Germany): Chimaira Buchhandelsgesellschaft; 2008. p. 186.

28. Upton SJ, McAllister CT, Freed PS, et al. *Cryptosporidium* spp. in wild and captive reptiles. J Wildl Dis 1989;25(1):20–30.
29. Caccio S. Molecular techniques to detect and identify protozoan parasites in the environment. Acta Microbiol Pol 2003;52(Suppl):23–34.
30. Griffin C, Reavill DR, Stacy BA, et al. Cryptosporidiosis caused by two distinct species in Russian tortoises and a pancake tortoise. Vet Parasitol 2010;170(1): 14–9.
31. Traversa D. Evidence for a new species of *Cryptosporidium* infecting tortoises: *Cryptosporidium ducismarci*. Parasit Vectors 2010;3(1):21.
32. Cranfield MR, Graczyk TK. Cryptosporidiosis. In: Mader WB, editor. Manual of reptile medicine and surgery. Philadelphia: W.B. Saunders Company, The Curtis Center; 1996. p. 359–63.
33. O'Donoghue PJ. *Cryptosporidium* and cryptosporidiosis in man and animals. Int J Parasitol 1995;25(2):139–95.
34. Graczyk TK, Cranfield MR. Experimental transmission of *Cryptosporidium* oocyst isolates from mammals, birds and reptiles to captive snake. Vet Res 1998;29: 187–95.
35. Fayer R. Taxonomy and species delimitation in *Cryptosporidium*. Exp Parasitol 2010;124(1):90–7.
36. Nowak MA, May RM. Superinfection and the evolution of parasite virulence. Proc Biol Sci 1994;255(1342):81–9.
37. Graczyk TK. Cryptosporidiosis in reptiles. Proceedings of the 7th International Symposium on Pathology and Medicine in Reptiles and Amphibians. Edition Chimaira. Berlin, 2004. p. 77–81.
38. Morita S, Namikoshi A, Hirata T, et al. Efficacy of UV irradiation in inactivating *Cryptosporidium parvum* oocysts. Appl Environ Microbiol 2002;68(11): 5387–93.
39. Carpenter C, Fayer R, Trout J, et al. Chlorine disinfection of recreational water for *Cryptosporidium parvum*. Emerg Infect Dis 1999;5(4):579.
40. Finch GR, Black EK, Gyürk L, et al. Ozone inactivation of *Cryptosporidium parvum* in demand-free phosphate buffer determined by in vitro excystation and animal infectivity. Appl Environ Microbiol 1993;59(12):4203–10.
41. Rataj AV, Lindtner-Knific R, Vlahović K, et al. Parasites in pet reptiles. Acta Vet Scand 2011;53(1):1–21.
42. Huang P, Weber JT, Sosin DM, et al. The first reported outbreak of diarrheal illness associated with *Cyclospora* in the United States. Ann Intern Med 1995; 123(6):409–14.
43. Duszynski DW, Steve JU, Lee C. Coccidia (Eimeria and Isospora) of Sauria. Available at: http://biology.unm.edu/biology/coccidia/sauria.html.
44. Isler CM, Bellamy JE, Wobeser GA. Labile neurotoxin in serum of calves with "nervous" coccidiosis. Can J Vet Res 1987;51:253–60.
45. Couch L, Stone PA, Duszynski DW, et al. A survey of the coccidian parasites of reptiles from islands of the Galápagos Archipelago: 1990-1994. J Parasitol 1996;82(3):432–7.
46. Sloboda M, Modrý D. New species of *Choleoeimeria* (Apicomplexa: *Eimeriidae*) from the veiled chameleon, *Chamaeleo calyptratus* (Sauria: *Chamaeleonidae*), with taxonomic revision of eimerian coccidia from chameleons. Folia Parasitol 2006;53(2):91–7.
47. McAllister CT. A new species of *Choleoeimeria* (Apicomplexa: *Eimeriidae*) from Oustalet's chameleon, *Furcifer oustaleti* (Sauria: *Chamaeleonidae*). Folia Parasitol 2012;59(1):12.

48. Paperna I, Lainson R. Ultrastructural study of meronts and gamonts of *Choleoeimeria rochalimai* (Apicomplexa: *Eimeriidae*) developing in the gall bladder of the gecko *Hemidactylus mabouia* from Brazil. Folia Parasitol 2000;47(2):91–6.

49. Abdel-Baki AS, El-Fayomi HM, Sakran T, et al. *Choleoeimeria saqanqouri* sp. nov. (Apicomplexa: *Eimeriidae*) infecting the gallbladder of *Scincus scincus scincus* (Reptilia: *Scincidae*) from Egypt. Acta Protozool 2008;47(2):143.

50. Lainson R. Some coccidial parasites of the lizard *Amphisbaena alba* (Reptilia: Amphisbaenia: *Amphisbaenidae*). Mem Inst Oswaldo Cruz 2003;98(7):927–36.

51. Matuschka FR. *Caryospora najae* sp. n. (Apicomplexa: *Sporozoea, Eimeriidae*) from the spitting cobra, *Naja nigricollis pallida* (Serpentes: Elapidae). J Parasitol 1982;68:1149–53.

52. Upton SJ, Current WL, Barnard SM. A new species of *Caryospora* (Apicomplexa: *Eimeriorina*) from *Elaphe* spp. (Serpentes: *Colubridae*) of the southeastern and central United States. Trans Am Microsc Soc 1984;103:240–4.

53. Matuschka FR. Reptiles as intermediate and/or final hosts of *Sarcosporidia*. Parasitol Res 1987;73(1):22–32.

54. Morsy K. *Sarcocystis acanthocolubri* sp. n. infecting three lizard species of the genus *Acanthodactylus* and the problem of host specificity. Light and electron microscopic study. Parasitol Res 2012;110(1):355–62.

55. Daszak P, Cunningham A. A report of intestinal sarcocystosis in the Bull snake (*Pituophis melanoleucus sayi*) and a reevaluation of *Sarcocystis* sp. from snakes of the genus *Pituophus*. J Wildl Dis 1995;31(3):400–3.

56. Eichinger D. Encystation in parasitic protozoa. Curr Opin Microbiol 2001;4(4):421–6.

57. Adam RD. The biology of *Giardia* spp. Microbiol Rev 1991;55(4):706.

58. Mader DR. Reptile medicine and surgery. St. Louis (MO): Elsevier Health Sciences; 2005.

59. Wolff ED, Salisbury SW, Horner JR, et al. Common avian infection plagued the tyrant dinosaurs. PLoS One 2009;4(9):e7288.

60. Borst GH, Vroege C, Poelma FG, et al. Pathological findings on animals in the Royal Zoological Gardens of the Rotterdam Zoo during the years 1963, 1964 and 1965. Acta Zool Pathol Antverp 1972;56:3.

61. Bhatt R, Abraham M, Petrin D, et al. New concepts in the diagnosis and pathogenesis of *Trichomonas vaginalis*. Can J Infect Dis 1996;7(5):321–5.

62. Vilela FC, da Silva MG, Barrella TH, et al. Trichomoniasis in *Bothrops jararaca* (Serpentes: *Viperidae*). J Venom Anim Toxins Incl Trop Dis 2003;9(1):105–10.

63. Richter B, Kübber-Heiss A, Weissenböck H, et al. Detection of *Cryptosporidium* spp., *Entamoeba* spp. and *Monocercomonas* spp. in the gastrointestinal tract of snakes by in-situ hybridization. J Comp Pathol 2008;138:63–71.

64. Barnard SM, Upton SJ. A veterinary guide to the parasites of reptiles. Volume 1: protozoa. Melbourne (FL): Krieger Publishing Company; 1994. p. 19–23.

65. Cooper JE, Jackson OF. Diseases of the reptilia, vol. 2. New York: Academic Press Inc (London) Ltd; 1981. p. 243–4.

66. Brugerolle G, Silva-Neto ID, Pellens R, et al. Electron microscopic identification of the intestinal protozoan flagellates of the xylophagous cockroach *Parasphaeria boleiriana* from Brazil. Parasitol Res 2003;90(3):249–56.

67. Jacobson E, editor. Infectious diseases and pathology of reptiles: color atlas and text. Boca Raton (FL): CRC Press; 2010. p. 574–5, 580–581.

68. Cooper JE, Jackson OF. Diseases of the reptilia, vols. 1–2. New York: Academic Press Inc (London) Ltd; 1981. p. 238–41.

69. Zwart P, Truyens EH. Hexamitiasis in tortoises. Vet Parasitol 1975;1(2):175–83.
70. Schneller P, Pantchev N. Parasitology in snakes, lizards and chelonians: a husbandry guide. Frankfurt am Main: Edition Chimaira. 2008. p. 32, 154, 165–73.
71. Zhang N, Suh S, Blackwell M. Microorganisms in the gut of beetles: evidence from molecular cloning. J Invertebr Pathol 2003;84(3):226–33.
72. Barrow JH, Stockton JJ. The influences of temperature on the host-parasite relationships of several species of snakes infected with *Entamoeba invadens*. J Eukaryot Microbiol 1960;7(4):377–83.
73. Teow WL, Ng GC, Chan PP, et al. A survey of *Blastocystis* in reptiles. Parasitol Res 1992;78(5):453–5.
74. Zierdt CH. *Blastocystis hominis*—past and future. Clin Microbiol Rev 1991;4(1):61.
75. Noël C, Dufernez F, Gerbod D, et al. Molecular phylogenies of *Blastocystis* isolates from different hosts: implications for genetic diversity, identification of species, and zoonosis. J Clin Microbiol 2005;43(1):348–55.
76. Satorhelyi T, Sreter T. Studies on internal parasites of tortoises. Parasitol Hung 1993;26:51–5.
77. Gartrell BD, Hare KM. Mycotic dermatitis with digital gangrene and osteomyelitis, and protozoal intestinal parasitism in Marlborough green geckos (*Naultinus manukanus*). N Z Vet J 2005;53(5):363–7.
78. Galavíz-Silva L, Jiménez-Guzmán F. *Zelleriella bayonai* n. sp. and *Nyctotherus uscae* n. sp. (Protozoa) from *Leptodeira maculata* (Colubridae) of Guatemala, C.A. Rev Biol Trop 1986;34(2):237–42.
79. Jacobson ER, Green DE, Undeen AH, et al. Systemic microsporidiosis in inland bearded dragons (*Pogona vitticeps*). J Zoo Wildl Med 1998;29:315–23.
80. Richter B, Csokai J, Graner I, et al. Encephalitozoonosis in two inland bearded dragons (*Pogona vitticeps*). J Comp Pathol 2013;148(2–3):278–82.
81. Coccidia of the world website. Available at: http://www.biology.unm.edu/biology/coccidia/home.html. Accessed 2013.
82. Gardner BB, Del Junco DJ, Fenn J, et al. Comparison of direct wet mount and trichrome staining techniques for detecting *Entamoeba* species trophozoites in stools. J Clin Microbiol 1980;12(5):656–8.
83. Kojimoto A, Uchida K, Horii Y, et al. Amebiasis in four ball pythons (*Python regius*). J Vet Med Sci 2001;63(12):1365–8.
84. Innis CJ, Garner MM, Johnson AJ, et al. Antemortem diagnosis and characterization of nasal intranuclear coccidiosis in Sulawesi tortoises (*Indotestudo forsteni*). J Vet Diagn Invest 2007;19(6):660–7.
85. Xiao L, Morgan UM, Limor J, et al. Genetic diversity within *Cryptosporidium parvum* and related *Cryptosporidium* species. Appl Environ Microbiol 1999;65(8):3386–91.
86. Spano F, Putignani L, McLauchlin J, et al. PCR-RFLP analysis of the *Cryptosporidium* oocyst wall protein (COWP) gene discriminates between *C. wrairi* and *C. parvum*, and between *C. parvum* isolates of human and animal origin. FEMS Microbiol Lett 1997;150(2):209–17.
87. Hopkins RM, Meloni BP, Groth DM, et al. Ribosomal RNA sequencing reveals differences between the genotypes of *Giardia* isolates recovered from humans and dogs living in the same locality. J Parasitol 1997;83:44–51.
88. Monis PT, Andrews RH, Mayrhofer G, et al. Molecular systematics of the parasitic protozoan *Giardia intestinalis*. Mol Biol Evol 1999;16(9):1135–44.
89. Kimbell LM III, Miller DL, Chavez W, et al. Molecular analysis of the 18S rRNA gene of *Cryptosporidium serpentis* in a wild-caught corn snake (*Elaphe guttata guttata*) and a five-species restriction fragment length polymorphism-based

assay that can additionally discern *C. parvum* from *C. wrairi*. Appl Environ Microbiol 1999;65(12):5345–9.

90. Graczyk TK, Cranfield MR, Fayer R. A comparative assessment of direct fluorescence antibody, modified acid fast stain, and sucrose flotation techniques for detection of *Cryptosporidium serpentis* oocysts in snake fecal specimens. J Zoo Wildl Med 1995;26:396–402.

91. Richter B, Nedorost N, Maderner A, et al. Detection of *Cryptosporidium* species in feces or gastric contents from snakes and lizards as determined by polymerase chain reaction analysis and partial sequencing of the 18S ribosomal RNA gene. J Vet Diagn Invest 2011;23:430.

92. Pedraza-Diaz P, Ortega-Mora LM, Carrion BA, et al. Molecular characterisation of *Cryptosporidium* isolates from pet reptiles. Vet Parasitol 2009;160: 204–10.

93. Research Associates Laboratories. Available at: www.vetdna.com. Accessed 2013.

94. Cerveny SN, Garner MM, D'Agostino JJ, et al. Evaluation of gastroscopic biopsy for diagnosis of *Cryptosporidium* sp. infection in snakes. J Zoo Wildl Med 2012; 43(4):864–71.

95. Royal Pharmaceutical Society of Great Britain. British national formulary. No. 44. London: BMJ Books; 2002.

96. Plumb DC. Plumb's veterinary drug handbook. Stockholm (WI): Pharma Vet Inc; 2005.

97. Brunton LL, Lazo JS, Parker KL. Goodman & Gilman's the pharmacological basis of therapeutics. 11th edition. New York: McGraw-Hill; 2006.

98. Gibbon PM, Klaphake E, Carpenter JW. Reptiles. In: Carpenter JW, Marion CJ, editors. Exotic animal formulary. 4th edition. St Louis (MO): Elsevier/Saunders; 2012. p. 83–182.

99. Funk RS, Diethelm G. Reptile formulary. In: Mader DR, editor. Reptile medicine and surgery. 2nd edition. St Louis (MO): Elsevier/Saunders; 2006. p. 1119–39.

100. Carpenter JW, Marion CJ, editors. Exotic animal formulary. 4th editiion. St Louis (MO): Elsevier/Saunders; 2012. p. viii.

101. Zimre-Grabensteiner E. Genetically different clonal isolates of *Trichomonas gallinae*, obtained from the same bird, can vary in their drug susceptibility, and *in vitro* evidence. Parasitol Int 2011;60(2):213–5.

102. Innis C, Papich M, Young D. Pharmacokinetics of metronidazole in the red-eared slider turtle (*Trachemys scripta elegans*) after single intracoelomic injection. J Vet Pharmacol Ther 2007;30(2):168–71.

103. Bodri MS, Rambo TM, Wagner RA, et al. Pharmacokinetics of metronidazole as a single oral bolus to red rat snakes. J Herpetol Med Surg 2006;16:15–9.

104. Iglesias R, Paramá A, Álvarez MF, et al. Antiprotozoals effective in vitro against the scuticociliate fish pathogen *Philasterides dicentrarchi*. Dis Aquat Org 2002; 49(3):191–7.

105. Clarke S, De-Gussem K, Barnes J. Flagellated protozoan infections in turkeys. World Poultry 2003;19(4):1–4.

106. Bogoslavsky BA. The use of ponazuril to treat coccidiosis in eight inland bearded dragons (*Pogona vitticeps*). Proc Ass Rep Amph Vet ARAV Fourteenth Annual Conference 2007. p. 8.

107. Modry D, Sloboda M. Control of coccidiosis in chameleons using toltrazuril—results of an experimental trial. Proceedings of the 7th International Symposium on Pathology and Medicine in Reptiles and Amphibians. Edition Chimaira. Berlin, 2004. p. 93–9.

108. Groza AM, Mederle N, Dărăbuş GH. Advocate—therapeutical solution in parasitical infestation in frillneck lizard (*Chalmydosaurus kingii*) and bearded dragon (*Pogona vitticeps*). Lucrari Stiintifice-Universitatea de Stiinte Agricole a Banatului Timisoara, Medicina Veterinara 2009;42(1):105–8.

109. Praschag P, Gibbons P, Boyer T, et al. An outbreak of intranuclear coccidiosis in *Pyxis* spp. tortoises. Proc 8th Annu Symp Conserv Biol Tortoises Freshwater Turtles. 2010. p. 42–3.

110. Katiyar SK, Gordon VR, McLaughlin GL, et al. Antiprotozoal activities of benzimidazoles and correlations with beta-tubulin sequence. Antimicrobial Agents Chemother 1994;38(9):2086–90.

111. Zajac AM, LaBranche TP, Donoghue AR, et al. Efficacy of fenbendazole in the treatment of experimental *Giardia* infection in dogs. Am J Vet Res 1998;59(1):61.

112. Cranfield MR, Graczyk TK. Cryptosporidiosis. In: Mader DR, editor. Reptile medicine and surgery. 2nd edition. St Louis (MO): Elsevier/Saunders; 2006. p. 756–62.

113. Coke RL, Tristan TE. *Cryptosporidium* infection in a colony of leopard geckos, *Euplepharis macularius*. Proc Annu Conf Rept Amph Vet 1998;157–63.

114. Fox LM, Saravolatz LD. Nitazoxanide: a new thiazolide antiparasitic agent. Clin Infect Dis 2005;40(8):1173–80.

115. Schnyder M, Kohler L, Hemphill A, et al. Prophylactic and therapeutic efficacy of nitazoxanide against *Cryptosporidium parvum* in experimentally challenged neonatal calves. Vet Parasitol 2009;160(1):149–54.

116. Pantchev N, Rushoff B, Kamhuber-Pohl A, et al. Kryptosporidiose-Therapie bei Leopardgeckos (*Eublepharis macularius*) mit Azithromycin (Zithromax®) und Paromomycinsulfat (Humatin®) – Fallbeispiele und Review der Literatur. Kleintierpraxis 2008;53(2):95–104.

117. Roberts CW, Roberts F, Henriquez FL, et al. Evidence for mitochondrial-derived alternative oxidase in the apicomplexan parasite *Cryptosporidium parvum*: a potential anti-microbial agent target. Int J Parasitol 2004;34(3):297–308.

118. Sen N, Majumder HK. Mitochondrion of protozoan parasite emerges as potent therapeutic target: exciting drugs are on the horizon. Curr Pharm Des 2008; 14(9):839–46.

119. Yabu Y, Minagawa N, Kita K, et al. Oral and intraperitoneal treatment of *Trypanosoma brucei brucei* with a combination of ascofuranone and glycerol in mice. Parasitol Int 1998;47(2):131–7.

120. Suzuki T, Hashimoto T, Yabu Y, et al. Direct evidence for cyanide-insensitive quinol oxidase (alternative oxidase) in apicomplexan parasite *Cryptosporidium parvum*: phylogenetic and therapeutic implications. Biochem Biophys Res Commun 2004;313(4):1044–52.

Index

Note: Page numbers of article titles are in **boldface** type.

A

Accipitriformes, as raptor classification, 212
    pellet composition in, 215–216
Acid-fast staining, for GI parasite microscopy, in reptile, 283–284
Adenocarcinoma, gastric, in chinchilla, 148
    in gerbil, 148–149
    in rat, 160
Adenovirus, in GI tract, of raptor, 225
Aggression, food and, 244–245
Alimentary tract, of rabbit, anatomy and physiology of, 166–167
Allometric scaling, for daily caloric needs, of companion mammal, 186–187
    of raptor, 221
American Ornithologist Union (AOU), classification of raptors, 211–212
Amoebae, in GI tract, of reptile, 272, 278–279
Amphotericin B, for *Macrorhabdus ornithogaster,* in avians, 207
Amylase enzymes, in GI tract, of fish, 126–127
    of rabbit, 169
Anesthesia, for GI tract procedures, in companion mammal, 180–182
    in fish, 128–130
Anole, green, GI parasites in, 276–277
Anorexia, in reptile, 254–255, 258
    with GI parasites, 286
Antibiotic-associated colitis, in hamster, 152–153
Antibody titers, for GI parasites, in reptile, 284–285
Antifungals, for *Macrorhabdus ornithogaster,* in avians, 208
Antimicrobial therapy, for GI disease, in companion mammal, 183, 192
    for liver lobe torsion, in rabbit, 200
Antiparasitics, for helminths, in raptor, 223–224
    for protozoa, in reptile, 288–291
Anus, in GI tract, of fish, 124
    class-based differences of, 125–126
    of guinea pig, imperforate, 150
Apicomplexan organisms, in GI tract, of reptile, 272–275
Ascarids, in GI tract, of raptor, 223
Aspicularis spp., in GI tract, of mice, 156
Assist feeding, of companion mammal, for GI disease, 187–188
    of reptiles, 250–255
        food choice for, 250–251
        gavage tubes for, 252–253
        indwelling tubes for, 253–254
        mechanics of, 251–255

Vet Clin Exot Anim 17 (2014) 299–332
http://dx.doi.org/10.1016/S1094-9194(14)00020-6
1094-9194/14/$ – see front matter © 2014 Elsevier Inc. All rights reserved.

Moving?

Make sure your subscription moves with you!

To notify us of your new address, find your **Clinics Account Number** (located on your mailing label above your name), and contact customer service at:

Email: journalscustomerservice-usa@elsevier.com

800-654-2452 (subscribers in the U.S. & Canada)
314-447-8871 (subscribers outside of the U.S. & Canada)

Fax number: 314-447-8029

Elsevier Health Sciences Division
Subscription Customer Service
3251 Riverport Lane
Maryland Heights, MO 63043

*To ensure uninterrupted delivery of your subscription, please notify us at least 4 weeks in advance of move.

Printed and bound by CPI Group (UK) Ltd, Croydon, CR0 4YY

03/10/2024

01040489-0004